TAKE THE WELLNESS ROAD

TO YOUR HEALTH AND FITNESS

BY COL. (Ret) DONALD E. ALSBRO, Ed.D., CHES

*"If we could give every individual the right amount
of nourishment and exercise, not too little and not too much,
we would have found the safest way to health.*

— Hippocrates, cc 400 bc

**This book is not intended to be a substitute for professional health care.
Please see your doctor if you have any medical concerns.**

BOOK CREDITS:

Author: Donald E. Alsbro
Editor and Design: Sharon Alsbro
Formatting by Sarah Thomas
Cover Design by Rosemary Boyd

With assistance from: Evelyn Cole Kissinger,
Liz Emrich, Jeff Haebig, Cesar Soto, and Sue Fanaly

*Cartoons by Wellness Quest, © reprinted by permission of Dr. Jeff Haebig,
Rochester, MN

Published by:
RAINBOW WELLNESS, INC.
942 Sierra Dr.
Benton Harbor, MI 49022

Copyright ©2007
Donald E. Alsbro, Ed.D., CHES
942 Sierra Dr.
Benton Harbor, MI 49022

www.dumpyourplump.com

ISBN: 0-9711114-0-5

All Rights Reserved.
No part of this book may be reproduced in any form or by any means
without written permission from the author.

TABLE OF CONTENTS

THIS BOOK IS DEDICATED TO:

My dad whom I only knew for a short time, but who gave me many values,

My athletic coaches who taught me the value of discipline and teamwork,

My friends I met in the military and education,

And most of all to my wife, Sharon, who patiently and lovingly provided inspiration and technical guidance, and numerous rewrites! Thanks!!!!!

ABOUT THE AUTHOR

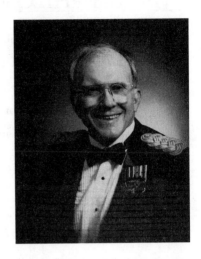

Dr. Don Alsbro graduated from Western Michigan University in 1963. In 1987, Don received his Doctoral Degree from Wayne State University. In 1991, he was designated as a Certified Health Education Specialist (CHES).

Dr. Alsbro retired as a Colonel from the U.S. Army after 31 years of service in the infantry, adjutant general and medical branches. His service included two tours in Vietnam and his last 15 years were spent as a hospital administrator. In 1991, Don was inducted into the Western Michigan University ROTC Alumni Hall of Fame.

Dr. Alsbro was a health and physical education instructor at Lake Michigan College in Benton Harbor, Michigan from 1973 to 1992. During this time, he developed the "Dump Your Plump™" program. Don was inducted into the Lake Michigan College's Athletic Hall of Fame in 2001.

Don enjoys competing in athletic events such as Senior Olympics and traveling with his wife Sharon. They have three grown, married children and especially enjoy spending time with them and their eight grandchildren.

MY PHILOSOPHY OF WELLNESS

- Daily exercise is NOT an option; it is a necessity.
- It's never too late to get the benefits of wellness.
- You will never FIND time for anything; you must MAKE it.
- The best exercise is the one you ENJOY and continue to do REGULARLY.
- Wellness is a LIFETIME activity.
- MIND, BODY and SPIRIT are inseparable.

The above statements summarize my wellness philosophy. Wellness is not easy, but it's worth it! There's an analogy that applies to wellness which deals with cost versus value. While the cost of physical wellness is relatively inexpensive, the value is immense.

History:

When I was in my twenties, I looked at "wellness" as physical fitness and chose activities that gave me "the most bang for the buck." Running could be done over the noon hour and still allow me to get back to the office. I was in the military and had to take a physical fitness test twice a year that consisted of push ups, sit ups, and the two mile run. Therefore, my fitness activities revolved around those activities. Also, we had to pass a semi annual body fat test. Wellness, to me meant physical fitness.

In my thirties and forties, I was still in the Army Reserves and taking fitness tests, but I was also teaching courses at the college such as: badminton, tennis, weight training, bowling, golf, racquetball, and running. Those are all activities that I enjoy doing in my free time, so I incorporated them in my fitness program. At this time, I also started teaching health classes and realized that fitness was a small, but important, part of wellness. I started thinking about the reduction of stress and eating right as cholesterol became a buzz word. I came to realize that wellness takes in the whole person. Optimal wellness is the process of improving a person's status in all dimensions, i.e. spiritual, mental and physical. WELLNESS TAKES INTO ACCOUNT THE WHOLE PERSON!

In my middle forties, I started experiencing hip pain, which at the age of 49 translated into a hip replacement. That meant that my fitness activities shifted to water aerobics, bicycling, and walking. I've always believed in the well-worn adage: "when life gives you lemons, make lemonade."

In my mid-fifties, I had my other hip replaced. People have asked why I had osteoarthritis and I truthfully can't answer. I don't have a weight problem. Possibly it could relate to an athletic injury from high school sports, badminton, tennis, or genetics.

Shortly after the second hip replacement, I was back to playing tennis, occasional badminton, swimming, weight training, fitness-walking, and table tennis. I've become involved in the Senior Olympic program and have won state honors in badminton and tennis. I also have learned to incorporate stretching into my fitness program and have taken steps to make changes in my lifestyle to include the other areas of wellness. I realize the importance of taking time for myself and my family, the importance of faith in a higher power and maintaining social contacts.

I give you my history to illustrate that if you make a lifetime commitment to wellness, as your physical capabilities change, you can change your activities. NEVER give up on the goal of wellness. "We're all signed up for life," so let's make the best of it!

Motivation:

I will never forget coming down the stairs as an eight-year-old and being told, "Now you are the man of the family." There's no question in my mind that my father's smoking, being over-weight, lack of exercise, and ignorance about nutrition were the major factors in his heart attack. Genetics may load the gun, but you have the choice whether or not to pull the trigger.

In the 1940's they didn't have the knowledge about smoking, nutrition, and exercise that we have today. With the knowledge we have today, there can be no excuse for indulging in these practices.

Wellness Pays Off!

In the three years that it's taken to write this book (I'm a slow writer), I've had quad-by-pass surgery, angioplasty (three times), a heart attack, and a pacemaker. However, I'm back to my fitness regimen. Thank goodness for modern medicine, but more importantly, thank goodness for my fitness regimen. With my inherited genetics for high cholesterol, homocysteine and c-reactive protein, I was a walking candidate for the same fate that befell my dad. But because of my exercise program, I had developed "collateral" circulation or extra pathways in the heart which enabled me to come through these ordeals with minimal damage. With the increased medical knowledge we now have and the lifestyle changes I have made, I look forward to the future and what it will bring.

YOU GOTTA START SOMEWHERE!!

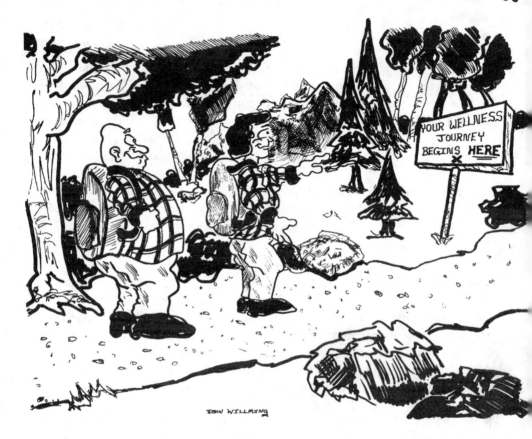

YOU CAN DO IT!
GOOD LUCK ON YOUR
WELLNESS JOURNEY!

— Don

MEDICAL HISTORY QUESTIONNAIRE

*If you answer **yes** to <u>any</u> of the following questions you are advised to seek medical approval prior to beginning an exercise program.*

	YES	NO
1. Are you a male over 40 or a female over 50 who is unaccustomed to vigorous activity?		
2. Have you ever had a heart attack?		
3. Has a doctor ever told you that you have high blood pressure, heart murmur, or heart or lung disease?		
4. Do you ever have chest, neck, shoulder or arm pains or pressure during or after exercise?		
5. Are you taking any medications for your heart?		
6. Do you frequently feel dizzy or have spells of severe dizziness?		
7. Have you recently had any acute infectious diseases?		
8. Have you had previous medical advice not to exercise?		
9. Do you have any joint problem that could be made worse by exercise?		
10. Do you have a family history of cardiovascular disease?		
11. Has it been more than three years since you had a medical check-up?		

The above questions are not intended to replace a medical evaluation. If you are at all concerned or if you answered YES to any of the questions, please see your physician before starting any fitness program. In most situations, the physician will give whole-hearted approval to becoming involved in a walking program.

"A medical examination is more urgent for those who plan to remain inactive than for those who intend to get into good physical shape."

— *Per-Olaf Astrand, M.D.*

WELLNESS INVENTORY ... *where do you stand?*

Take this health risk inventory prior to starting your wellness journey and then repeat the inventory at the end of the program. Each "no" answer indicates a personal health risk factor. The guidelines in this book can help you make the changes that will provide more "YES" answers in your life.

	PRE Y/N	POST Y/N
DATE		
FITNESS		
Do you exercise aerobically 3-5 times a week (at least 30 min./session)?		
Do you do muscle strengthening work at least twice a week?		
Do you perform stretching/flexibility exercises at least 3 times a week?		
WEIGHT CONTROL		
Do you know what your body fat percentage is?		
Do you know what your ideal weight should be?		
Are you presently within 5 lbs. of your ideal weight?		
NUTRITION		
Do you read labels before you purchase food products?		
Do you limit dietary fats (especially saturated fats)?		
Do you limit cholesterol in your diet?		
Do you limit sodium in your diet?		
Do you monitor your intake of sugars?		
Do you avoid low fiber, processed meals?		
Do you get at least 25 grams of fiber a day?		
Do you take a daily multi-vitamin?		

	PRE Y/N	POST Y/N
SMOKING AND ALCOHOL		
Are you a non-smoker?		
Do you know your alcohol limit?		
If you drink, do you limit yourself to 2 or less drinks a day?		
Do you refrain from driving after drinking?		
BLOOD PRESSURE/HEART RATE		
Is your blood pressure below 140/90?		
Do you have your blood pressure taken every 6-12 months?		
What is your resting heart-rate? (List)		
CHOLESTEROL		
Do you have your cholesterol level checked regularly?		
What is your total cholesterol? (List)		
What is your HDL (Good) Cholesterol? (List)		
If your total cholesterol is over 200, have you asked for an HDL/LDL ratio?		
STRESS		
Do you take time each day to relax?		
Do you take minor hassles in stride?		
Do you get enough sleep each night?		
SPIRITUALITY		
Do you regularly attend a worship service?		
Do you have a person you can seek spiritual advice from?		

We all remember the buddy system when we were growing up. We've all experienced the power of teams and how much more you can do as a team as opposed to working alone. As an example, one Clydesdale horse can pull up to a certain amount of weight, but when he's hitched to another Clydesdale, the team can pull 3-4 times the weight, instead of just double.

Teamwork Divides the Task and Doubles the Success!

Numerous studies have shown the power of the buddy system in the adult world, especially when trying to change a lifestyle behavior. During the Dump Your Plump™ and Movin' & Winnin' programs, I've observed that when the husband and wife are both involved, they are more likely to do better because they help each other. Study after study has shown that a person is much more likely to stick with an exercise program or a nutritional plan if there is social support. As one contestant who lost 25 pounds stated: "It's easy to let yourself down, but hard to let your team down."

Behavioral contracts encourage the development of social support when they are clearly defined and supportive in nature. On the next page is a "buddy" contract designed to help you make your exercise and weight goals. The public commitment increases the likelihood of persistence when obstacles occur.

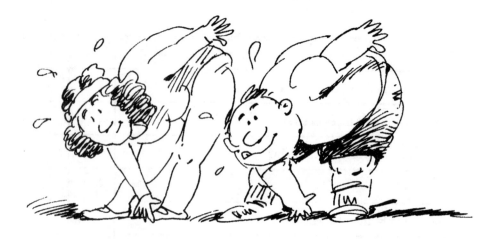

BUDDY CONTRACT

I, _____, pledge to meet the following goals:

    a._____

    b._____

    c._____

My buddy, who has signed the contract below, agrees to provide me with the following supportive actions:

    a._____

    b._____

    c._____

I will begin my program on: _____

I will finish on: _____

My wellness activities will be:

    <u>Activity:</u> _____ <u>Days of Week:</u>

    _____

    _____

My reward for making my goals: _____

I have entered into this contract under sound mind and body, and I am confident that I will make my goals.

Signed _____ Date _____

Supporting Buddy _____ Date _____

The nice feature of smorgasbords is that we can take as much or as little of an item as we want. If we don't like peas and carrots, we can take the broccoli and spinach instead. Or we can have two pieces of fish and skip the chicken or we can choose beans instead of meat. As our taste preferences change, we become more willing to sample those foods that we previously shunned.

That is the way I'd like you to approach this book. I've tried to give you a "smorgasbord" approach to wellness. I have included a wide range of topics from acupuncture (a) to yoga (y). Read the subjects that presently appeal to you and skip over the ones you are not ready for. Down the wellness road, you may decide that topics such as meditation, Qigong or yoga are ones that you'd like to learn more about. I remember when I used to pick up the health magazines and search out the fitness articles and skip over the rest. Now, I still look for the fitness, but I also read about nutrition, supplementation, and alternative medicine.

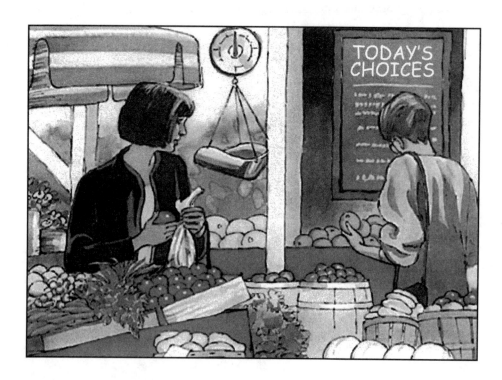

CHAPTER ONE:
YOUR WELLNESS JOURNEY

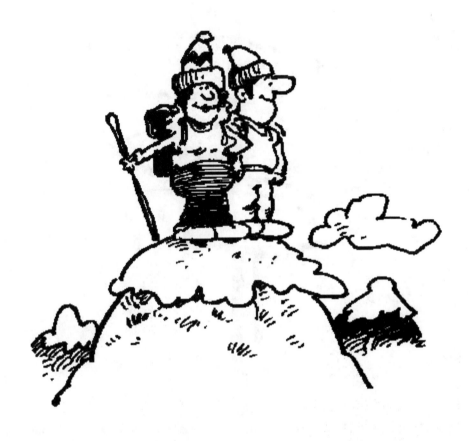

You do not need anyone's permission to empower yourself to be responsible for your health. Take action! Even if it means temporary discomfort and inconvenience. Your life depends on it!

— Don Alsbro

YOU CAN'T GET ANYWHERE UNTIL YOU START!

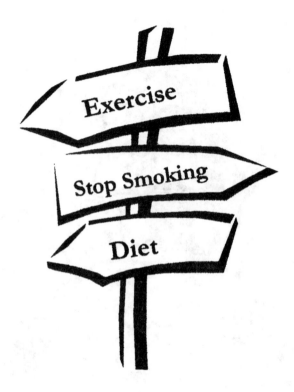

What is wellness? What is health? Are they the same? Many people assume that good health is simply the absence of physical disease. A majority of people tend to consider themselves to be in "good health," yet we know from national statistics that 60-70% need to improve their health habits. Less than 20% exercise the recommended amount, up to 50% are overweight, and over 30% still smoke.

Wellness is an active process of becoming aware and making choices toward a healthier life. Wellness defines the movement toward an advanced state of health, or "high level health." The relationship can be much clearer if we view health as existing on a continuum.

> *"Health is the first wealth."*
> *— Ralph Waldo Emerson*

ILLNESS / WELLNESS MODEL

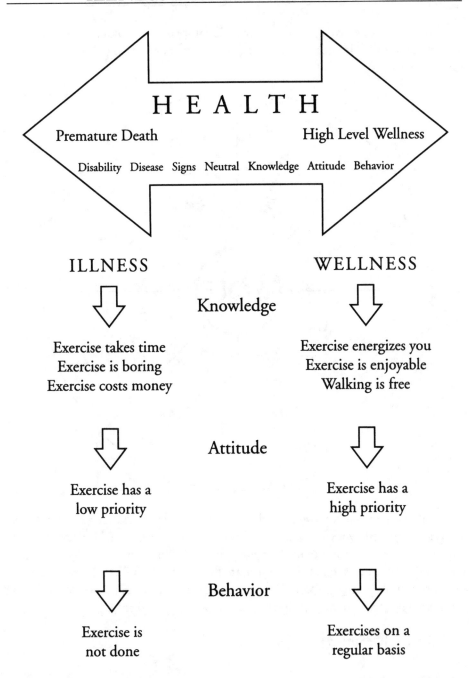

H E A L T H

Premature Death   High Level Wellness

Disability Disease Signs Neutral Knowledge Attitude Behavior

ILLNESS   WELLNESS

Knowledge

Exercise takes time   Exercise energizes you
Exercise is boring   Exercise is enjoyable
Exercise costs money   Walking is free

Attitude

Exercise has a   Exercise has a
low priority   high priority

Behavior

Exercise is   Exercises on a
not done   regular basis

WHICH SIDE ARE YOU ON?
(Alsbro, p. 2)

WELLNESS is an active process of becoming aware of and making choices toward a more successful existence. Wellness is achieved by making progress in these seven interrelated areas:

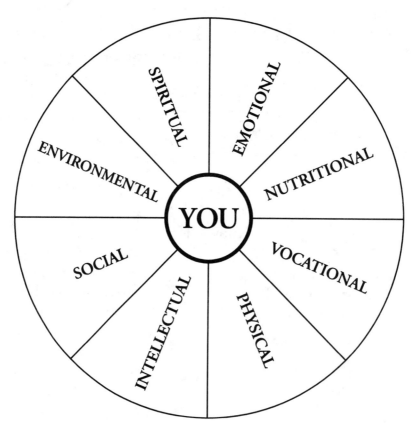

It should be understood that you could exhibit high level wellness in one or two areas, such as physical and vocational, but low level wellness in the others. No one is at the same place on the continuum in all six areas. Even within the physical area, there are the sub-components, such as aerobics, strength, weight, flexibility and medical self-responsibility. An individual could be a regular exerciser, but exhibit poor nutritional skills or demonstrate unhealthy habits such as, smoking or drinking.

WHAT CHOICES ARE YOU MAKING?

THE GOAL IS:
BALANCE!

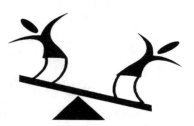

Change can be difficult, and it can be threatening. It involves looking hard at oneself and making a decision to take action. Failure is a possibility. Motivational speaker Zig Ziglar says, "So what! Failure is an event, not a person!" Abraham Lincoln, Thomas Edison, Henry Ford, Walt Disney, and Babe Ruth all had failures, but their successes are remembered.

A "magic pill" to take off weight, stop smoking, or exercise the body would be ideal. The reality is that people must make the effort themselves to achieve permanent change. There is no "magic pill."

A good phrase to keep in mind is, "If the mind can conceive and believe it, the body can achieve it." Picture yourself ten weeks from now making your weight goal and exercising daily. If you can visualize that, chances are you will accomplish it.

> "I've missed more than 9,000 shots in my career. I've lost almost 300 games. Twenty-six times, I've been trusted to take the game winning shot and missed. I've failed over and over and over again in my life. And that is why I succeed!"
>
> — *Michael Jordan*
> *(Selected the greatest athlete of the 20th century!)*

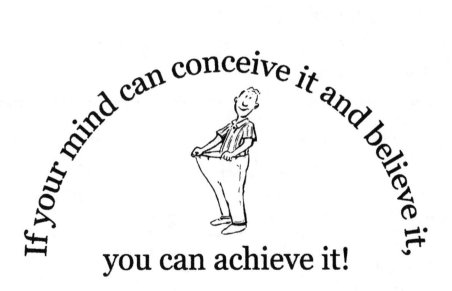

If your mind can conceive it and believe it, you can achieve it!

STAGES OF CHANGE (Spiral Model)

The "Stages of Change" Transtheoretical Model developed by Dr. James Prochaska offers insight into how behaviors are changed. Dr. Prochaska states that change in human behavior is simply a point on a continuum that is spiral, not linear; thus there is no such thing as failure. He says there are five stages: pre-contemplation, contemplation, preparation, action, and maintenance. (Prochaska)

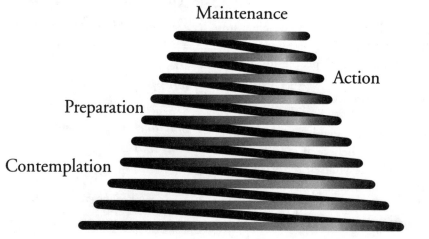

Maintenance

Action

Preparation

Contemplation

Pre-contemplation

Pre-contemplation: *"Get off my back."*   *"I don't have a problem!"*

We start out thinking such thoughts about exercising, losing weight or quitting smoking.

- *"I don't need to exercise. I have enough energy to do my job."*
- *"I don't think about losing weight. I like eating, and besides, I don't think it's a problem."*
- *"Smoking doesn't bother me. We all have to die from something. If it wasn't smoking, it would be something else."*

Do these statements sound familiar? People in this phase are either unaware that they have a problem or are unwilling to recognize it. They don't believe that the negative aspects of the behavior outweigh the positive aspects. In other words, people won't change until the pain not to change exceeds the pain to change. They cannot move forward until they acknowledge there is a problem and "take ownership" of it.

"LIFE IS CHANGE – GROWTH IS OPTIONAL"
— Karen Kaiser Clark

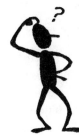

Contemplation:

"I'm thinking about it."   *"Maybe I do have a problem."*

If you've already decided to begin a program, then you have already moved from the pre-contemplation phase to the contemplation, and your chances of success have improved immeasurably.

Preparation:

"I'm going to start exercising next week."
"I'm going to start a food diary next week."

You know when you'll start and you have begun to prepare for it. You've gone public by informing your friends and now you have started to select your weight and exercise goals. In this stage, a person is planning to take action in the very near future.

Action:

"I'm exercising five times a week. "I've hidden the television remote."
"I'm watching my serving sizes and fat calories."
"I will eat breakfast so that my metabolism will get a jump start."

This is the "doing" phase, and you will be in this phase for a long time, hopefully for the rest of your life. Be aware of the pitfalls and have strategies to prevent relapses.

Maintenance:

"I look forward to my daily exercise."
"I have more energy and enjoy receiving compliments on how good I look."
"I have learned to make better food choices."

Maintenance is getting used to a new habit. This stage requires hard work to keep the desired behavior change. It is a long, ongoing process, usually with relapses. Learn from the relapses and keep moving forward. Remember it is not easy, but it is worthwhile! Keep up this new behavior for at least a year and you will have become a new person.

CONGRATULATIONS!

LAPSE, RELAPSE OR COLLAPSE?

According to Dr. Prochaska, "Linear progression is possible but a relatively rare phenomenon, especially with addictive behaviors." We all know that it may take several attempts to change an eating behavior or to stop smoking. There are many things you can learn from a lapse or relapse. You may not have budgeted enough time, perhaps stressful events occurred during the program, or perhaps you didn't take full advantage of the strategies available to you, such as outside support, rewards, etc.

This is not the time to abandon the project. You've already determined that eliminating the behavior will produce dividends down the road. Evaluate where you've progressed on the Stages of Change model and look to avoid the people, situations, and objections that led you astray. At the same time, adhere closely to those people and situations that gave you strength.

> ## Don't let a LAPSE turn into a RELAPSE and then into a COLLAPSE!

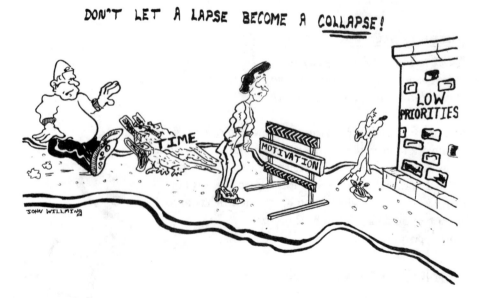

AN AUTOBIOGRAPHY IN FIVE CHAPTERS

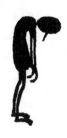

CHAPTER ONE
I walk down the street.
There's a deep hole in the sidewalk.
I fall in.
I'm lost. I'm helpless.
It isn't my fault.
It takes forever to find a way out.

CHAPTER TWO
I walk down the street.
There's a deep hole in the sidewalk.
I pretend I don't see it.
I fall in, again.
I can't believe I'm in the same place.
But it isn't my fault.
It still takes a long time to get out.

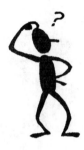

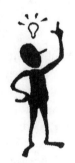

CHAPTER THREE
I walk down the same street.
There's a deep hole in the sidewalk.
I see it's there.
I fall in … it's a habit … but my eyes are open.
I know where I am.
It's my fault.
I get out immediately.

CHAPTER FOUR
I walk down the same street.
There's a deep hole in the sidewalk.
I walk around it.

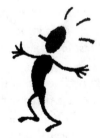

CHAPTER FIVE
I walk down a different street!

Author Anonymous

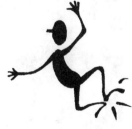

WHAT STREET ARE YOU WALKING DOWN?

GENETICS OR ENVIRONMENT?

"GENETICS PERMIT OBESITY, BUT ENVIRONMENT CREATES IT."
Kelley Brownell, noted weight management authority,
at a national health conference

TOXIC ENVIRONMENT!! This may be upsetting to some individuals, but our health problems, particularly weight problems, aren't a result of genetics but rather CHOICES!

> *"I strongly believe when the Creator designed our body, it was designed to hunt, fish, run, walk, jump, in other words, to MOVE! We wouldn't have a weight problem in this country if we didn't first have a movement problem."*
>
> — *Don Alsbro, Founder of Dump Your Plump™*

Heart disease, Type II diabetes, depression, certain cancers, and many other chronic diseases are mainly lifestyle related. Prior to the 1950's, we were a much more manual society. Families had only one car; kids walked or rode bicycles to school; after school activities were active and outside; lawns were mowed by push mowers; snow was shoveled manually; wood was chopped; lawns were raked; gardens were hoed; lawns were watered by hand; the golf course was walked; cars had manual transmissions; garage doors were opened manually; typewriters were manual; television was in its infancy, and remote controls hadn't been invented; cellular phones were nonexistent; and fast food hadn't even been thought of.

Did you know that the remote control has added seven pounds of fat PER year to the average person's body? The average person watches or listens to over five hours a day of TV. Prior to the remote, viewers would get up to change the TV fifteen times during the day. The personal computer is another example of added pounds because of technology. The manual typewriter required 20 calories per hour more to operate than today's word processor. If a secretary types six hours a day, 5 days a week, 50 weeks a year, this adds up to seven pounds gained PER year.

FOUR AGES OF MAN: *The only thing that changes is the distance from the TV.*

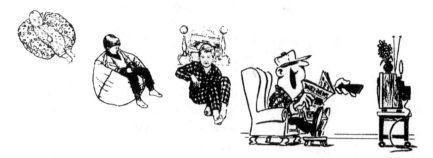

FACT: **Adults watch 40 hours a week of TV, adolescents 24 hours. T.V. stands for "Time Vacuum."**

There is a direct relationship between TV and obesity. The same relationship of choices occurs when it comes to nutrition. In the 50's, the average grocery store had 5,000 items; today there are over 32,000 items, and the list grows every day. Food manufacturers have found a way to preserve food life (not human life) by adding hydrogen, palm oil, and coconut oil to our foods. In the 50's, only 5% of our meals were eaten out. Today over 50% of the meals are eaten out, many of them at fast food restaurants, now on every street corner.

> REGULAR, MODERATE PHYSICAL ACTIVITY IS ONE OF THE BEST FORMS OF STRESS MANAGEMENT. IT IS INEXPENSIVE, LONG LASTING, EFFECTIVE AND FUN.

Another toxic environmental area is stress and the demands of our fast paced lifestyle. This is an area that is hard to measure, since what is stress to one person may be stimulating to another. Each of us has different stress levels, and when we reach these levels, we should be able to employ such stress relieving techniques as meditation, visualization, prayer, and exercise. Regular, moderate physical activity is one of the best forms of stress management. It is inexpensive, long lasting, effective, and FUN.

Should we throw out the remotes, snow blowers, garage door openers, cellular phones, etc? NO! The answer is that we must find other enjoyable ways to get in the activity we've lost.

DEFINITION OF LIFESTYLE:
A style of living that consistently reflects a particular set of values and attitudes

WHAT IS YOUR LIFESTYLE?

".... Two roads diverged in a wood, and I – I took the one less traveled by. And that has made all the difference."

"The Road Not Taken" by Robert Frost

Using Robert Frost's analogy, you're at a fork in the road: one path travels downhill and has obviously been heavily traveled, while the other rises slowly uphill to great heights. Will you take the easy route or be motivated to take the high road and enjoy the beauty from above? All the events of your life have led up to the moment where your roads diverge and you must choose your road. Choose wisely!

> *"I have a favorite saying: "You can pay a small price now, or pay a big price later." There is a well-known oil filter company that advertises that slogan on the side of their trucks. In regards to your car, you can change your oil on a regular basis or pay for a new engine later. When it comes to our bodies, we can do some daily exercise and live a long, quality life or we can be a couch potato and take our chances. Unfortunately, we can't buy new bodies. We are given one body and the CHOICES we make today will determine our future!"*
>
> —Don Alsbro

Many people have chosen the easy route, and consequently the United States has become the fattest nation in the world. We also lead the world in heart and lung disease, as well as cancer and diabetes. Diabetes has increased 700% since World War II! The goal of the author is to convince America to take the high road of exercise and eating sensibly. It will make all the difference in the world!

What is the high road? It is an active lifestyle based upon at least 30 minutes of daily activity; abstaining from tobacco and drugs, moderate or no use of alcohol; making sensible nutritional choices (that doesn't mean dieting-there is no such thing as a bad food-just inappropriate choices and amounts); using your seat belt; getting adequate rest; eating regular meals, including a good healthy breakfast; including humor in your life; and maintaining close relationships. These all seem easy to do, but unfortunately, they seem to be on that less traveled road.

As I have moved down the road, I hope that I've taken the road less traveled, and in the process have taken along a few fellow travelers. I would consider my life to be a failure if, when my house of flesh and bone is gone, that I had not touched at least one person's life!

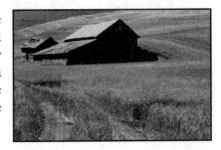

A famous study of octogenarians, conducted in the 70's by Dr. Lester Breslow of the UCLA School of Public Health, concluded that by following these seven health habits, men could add eleven years to their lives and women seven years:

- Regular exercise
- Adequate sleep
- Good breakfast
- Regular meals
- Weight control
- Abstaining from tobacco and drugs
- Moderate or zero use of alcohol

A more recent study by Michael F. Roizen, MD and three other scientists in the best seller Real Age (Roizen, 1999), evaluated 25,000 medical studies and determined 126 health behaviors that influence our rate of aging. He compared a person's calendar age (actual age), to his biological age. Thus a person could be 40 years old and have a body age of 30, or 60, depending upon his lifestyle and genetics. According to Dr. Roizen, inherited genetics accounts for less than 30% of all aging effects. Dr. Roizen has outlined 44 steps that will delay aging; some are relatively easy and others are harder.

TAKE THE REAL AGE
QUIZ ON LINE:
www.RealAge.com

The quiz takes approximately 30 minutes and requires personal data such as cholesterol, blood pressure, weight, vitamins, etc. It will calculate what your Real Age would be if you adopted appropriate health behaviors.

In his new book **Real Age Makeover** (Roizen, 2004) Dr. Roizen (who's 58, but has a "real age" of 40), says "Most people can get eight to 12 years younger just by walking 30 minutes a day and changing two other small things, like taking aspirin daily or using 9" plates to control portion size."

He continues by giving his magic "real age" formula: clean arteries, a healthy immune system and smart living. This means exercise, eat right, take vitamins, don't smoke and wear your seat belt.

In the spring of 2004, the Center for Disease Control announced that deaths from inactivity and obesity have equaled deaths from smoking as the leading lifestyle cause of death. This number has risen from 300,000 in 1990 to 400,000 in 2000 and continues to grow.

"Whether you live one day longer is really not the ultimate goal. What is important is the quality of life ... A life that is happy, healthy, and productive."

— Kenneth H. Cooper, M.D.

GOALS

Know where you want to go,
so you'll know when you get there!

Without goals, you won't know where you're going or when you've arrived. What is the number one reason businesses fail? The reason 80% of businesses fail in their first five years is that they do not have a business plan, and if they have one, it is probably not realistic. You need a plan with realistic and flexible goals, short term, intermediate and long range goals You also need clearly defined time lines, cash flow projections, and strategies to overcome obstacles. In other words, it must be thoroughly thought out and researched.

The same idea applies to your exercise and weight loss program. Just going out and doing your 30 minutes a day with no plan doesn't bode well for long term success. We need to have a well-thought-out plan with realistic goals and strategies to accomplish these goals. As motivational speaker Zig Ziglar states, "Goals are nothing more than dreams with dates attached to them." For a goal to be useful, it must be specific, realistic, and flexible. Strive for goals YOU want to reach, not goals someone else sets for you.

But before you start writing your goals, you must do some introspection. You must decide who you're doing this for and WHY. You must be doing this for yourself and not to please a friend, spouse, or your doctor. Of course, if you have the support of your friends, spouse, and doctor, it will be much easier. You must have a why or a reason, and if it isn't big enough, you'll struggle. Put your goals on the refrigerator and bathroom mirrors where you'll see them daily.

For some people, their WHY is a "wake up" call. We all know people who were confirmed couch potatoes, with no interest in exercise, UNTIL they had their first heart attack. Then they became confirmed fitness addicts. Unfortunately for many people, their first heart attack is sudden death, and they don't have a second chance. Other's "wake up" call is not being able to put on the clothing that fit last year or preparing to attend a high school reunion, or being told by the doctor that unless you lose the weight, lower the blood pressure, etc. chances are good that you will not be around to see your children or grandchildren graduate from high school.

WHAT ARE YOUR PRIORITIES?

In truth, we can all find time to do something if it is important enough to us. The secret to fitting exercise into your life is to change your perspective on how you spend your time and to accept the value of allocating time for yourself.

Make sure that you are doing the program for yourself and not for someone or something else. The bottom line is if you have a WHY, then the WHAT, WHERE, WHEN, and the HOW will take care of itself.

Specific Goals:

Your goal must be measurable. Instead of vowing to "reduce fat" or "exercise more," write the what, when, where, and how of your goals. For example: "On Monday I will walk with my husband at 7 p.m. for 30 minutes at Patriot's Park."

Realistic Goals:

Realistic goals take into account where you are today and what you could accomplish with reasonable effort. Don't be a perfectionist; avoid goals that use the words, "always," "never," or "everyday."

Flexible Goals:

Modify your goals if necessary. They should be challenging, not overwhelming. That is why I strongly recommend at the beginning of a 10 week program, that you not select a 20 lb. goal. It's better to be successful at losing 10-15 lbs. than to be disappointed when you just miss your goal by a couple of pounds, yet you're in the best physical shape you've been for a long time.

Short Term Goals:

These would be daily or weekly goals. Motivational speaker Murry Banks, several years ago, won his age group for the Hawaiian Ironman Triathalon. This Triathalon combines swimming, bicycling, and running and is considered by many yo be the ultimate fitness challenge. Murray talks about how he didn't focus on the finish line during the race but rather each telephone pole on the route. When he got to that pole, he reset his goal to get to the next one, and eventually he got to the finish line.

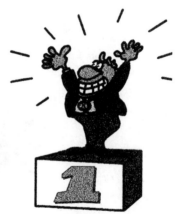

SETTING **SMART** GOALS. *Each goal should be...*
✓ Specific – the more detailed the better
✓ Measurable – need to know when the goal is attained.
✓ Attainable – is it physically and mentally possible?
✓ Realistic – is it a realistic goal?
✓ Timed – when is the deadline?

In weight loss, don't try to climb Mt. Everest in a 10 week program. We didn't get overweight and out of shape overnight. It will take a long time to get where we want to be. Maybe our long range goal is to lose 100 lbs. Set a short range goal to lose 25 lbs., and when you accomplish that goal, then re-set for another 25 lbs. It is easier to climb 4 small hills than to climb one giant hill. So what if you're only losing 2 lbs. a week. That translates into 100 lbs. in a year and if you lose the weight gradually through diet and exercise, the chances of keeping it off are much better than if you lost it in a shorter period. You're not losing lean body tissue or muscle, but rather fat.

Intermediate Goals:

These may be where you want to be at halfway through the program. This gives you an idea if your original long term goals were realistic. Just as athletes change their game plan at halftime of an athletic event, so should you evaluate if your goals need to be readjusted. As someone said, the goals remain the same, but the time frame changes.

Long Range Goals:

These are one year, five years and even lifetime goals. When we reach our long range goal, we need to congratulate ourselves (we did it — no one did it for us), take a short break, and then re-set our goals. We are either moving forward in life or backwards. There is no standing still!

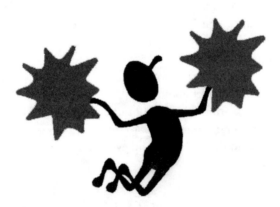

CELEBRATE YOUR ACHIEVEMENTS!!!

SAMPLE GOALS FOR A TEN WEEK WELLNESS PROGRAM

Short Term Goals (weekly)

- Exercise at least 5 times this week for at least 30 minutes a day.
- Make a nutritious choice at least one meal a day — for example, for lunch have a salad with fat free dressing, instead of a Big Mac.
- Make my weekly weight loss goal (1/10 of my 10 week goal).
- Support my buddy.
- Cut down on between meals snacking.

Intermediate Goals (half way through the 10 weeks)

- Exercise 25 days for 5 weeks (5 days each week).
- Make 60% of my weight loss goal.
- Make a nutritious choice at each meal.
- Exercise an additional 15-30 minutes once or twice a week.

Long Range Goals (completion of 10 weeks)

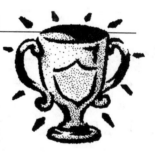

- Exercise 50 days out of 50.
- Make my weight goal.
- Continue to exercise and eat sensibly for a LIFETIME!
- Reward myself for completing the contest and being a WINNER!

MY ONE MINUTE WELLNESS ASSESSMENT

On a scale of 1 to 10, using your own definitions and current perspective, give yourself a score to indicate your present assessment of health for each factor.

1 = VERY UNHEALTHY; 10 = FULL HEALTH

MY PHYSICAL HEALTH		MY SOCIAL HEALTH	
MY EMOTIONAL HEALTH		MY FAMILY HEALTH	
MY SPIRITUAL HEALTH		MY WORK HEALTH	
MY INTELLECTUAL HEALTH		MY NUTRITIONAL HEALTH	

LONG TERM, INTERMEDIATE AND SHORT TERM GOALS

GOAL SHEET FOR _____

DATE: _____

Weekly Goals (Short Term)	Plan of Action	Rewards
_____		
_____		
_____		

Half Way Goals DATE: _____	Plan of Action	Rewards
_____		
_____		
_____		

Long Term Goal	Plan of Action	Rewards
_____		
_____		
_____		

Completion Date: _____

Post this goal sheet where you can see it on a daily basis, for example on your bathroom mirror, refrigerator, or in your daily planner.

CHAPTER TWO:
WHY LOSE WEIGHT?

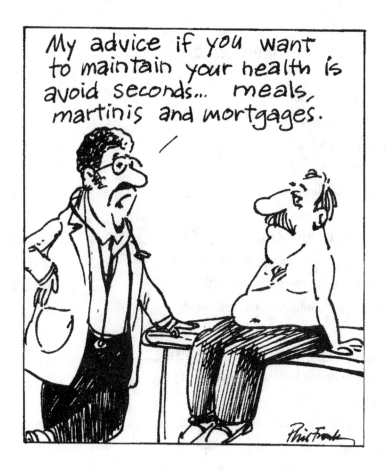

Want to Add Ten Years To Your Life?

Scientists at Loma Linda University conducted a study of 34,000 Seventh-Day Adventists. Their findings were "The Adventists who practiced healthy habits – eating a vegetarian diet, getting vigorous exercise, never smoked, maintaining a healthy weight, and eating nuts five times a week – lived a full ten years longer than those who did none of these things."

(Archives of Internal Medicine, 9 July 2001)

WHY LOSE WEIGHT?

You can pay the small price now (smart choices)
or you can pay the big price later (heart attack).

Excess weight contributes to:

- Heart disease
- Increased risk for cancer
- High blood pressure
- Increased risk for diabetes
- Increased risk for arthritis
- Increased back problems

Excess weight also contributes to:

- Lack of energy to travel or enjoy recreational activities
- Lack of energy to enjoy family and friends
- Decreased self-confidence and self-esteem

Losing excess weight contributes to:

- Decrease in health and life insurance costs.
- Increased energy
- Longer life: obesity-decreasing exercise can increase your life span by seven years
- Better sleep
- Better ability to deal with stress
- and on, and on, and on, and......

BOTTOM LINE: YOU'LL LOOK AND FEEL BETTER.

Should I Lose Weight?

Kenneth Cooper, MD, the "Father of Aerobics," suggests the pride test:
"Do you like what you see when you stand naked in front of a mirror?

HOW MUCH OF YOU IS FAT?
WHY DOES IT MATTER?

Because weight can be misleading, you need to know your body composition. The purpose of the test is to determine how much of your body is composed of fat and how much is lean body tissue. If you score a 20 percent on the body-fat test, it means that 20 percent of your weight is composed of fat.

Weight is a very personal issue with most people. Your focus should be on exercise. If you exercise on a daily basis and eat sensibly (NOT DIET), you will not have a weight problem, unless you have a medical problem.

A scale can be very misleading and your weight, per se, is of limited value. Your weight is the grand total of your bones, organs, blood, fat, muscle, and other tissue. Since muscle weighs more than fat (122% more), the scale weight can be misleading. Consider two men who stand 5'11" and both weigh 190 lbs. One is an active person who weight trains, plays tennis and badminton, swims, and power walks. He is considered fit. The other man is a couch potato whose stomach hangs four inches over his belt buckle, and the most strenuous exercise he does is exercising the trigger finger on the TV remote. So you can see that even though these two are the same height and weight, the first can register 15% body fat (excellent) and the latter registers 30% (obese). It is important to know how much of the body weight is fat and how much is muscle. The scales don't give this breakdown. Thus, the best measurement is the body fat test.

Why use the scales at all if it is misleading? The answer: it is the easiest assessment tool available. If you understand the limitations of scales, then you can use some common sense interpreting the figures. It is important to have a goal or target to aim for, and weighing in keeps you focused.

Body fat is more than a cosmetic measure; it can have serious health implications. According to Dr. Roizen in Real Age, being overweight can provoke many conditions that age your body. According to his calculations, being overweight can make your Real Age as much as ten years older than your chronological age.

Having too little fat can cause problems, too. This usually affects women more than men. For women, a super-low body fat, generally below 12%, can lead to irregular menstrual periods, permanent bone loss, and a high rate of bone fractures.

Why do we do body-fat testing?

Our body composition falls into 2 categories. One is lean body mass, which makes muscles, bone, organs and water. The other category is fat. Using a bathroom scale does not indicate how fat a person is because both fat and lean body mass contribute to the total weight.

BODY FAT CLASSIFICATIONS

Body Fat Percentages:
(Based on National Institute of Health/BMI Guidelines)

WOMEN

Age	Ideal %	Good %	Moderate %	Fat %	Obese %
<19	17	17.5-22	22.5-27	27.5-32	32.5+
20-29	18	18.5-23	23.5-28	28.5-33	33.5+
30-39	19	19.5-24	24.5-29	29.5-34	34.5+
40-49	20	20.5-25	25.5-30	30.5-35	35.5+
50+	21	21.5-26	26.5-31	31.5-36	36.5+

MEN

Age	Ideal %	Good %	Moderate %	Fat %	Obese %
<19	12	12.5-17	17.5-22	22.5-27	27.5+
20-29	13	13.5-18	18.5-23	23.5-28	28.5+
30-39	14	14.5-19	19.5-24	24.5-29	29.5+
40-49	15	15.5-20	20.5-25	25.5-30	30.5+
50+	16	16.5-21.5	21.5-26	26.5-31	31.5+

REMEMBER: It's fat, not necessarily the number on a scale, that puts us at risk for heart disease, high blood pressure, some cancers, low self-esteem, etc., etc....

"One should eat to live, not live to eat."
— Jean Baptiste Moliere

CAUTIONS IN THE APPLICATION
OF BODY FAT PERCENTAGES

While experts haven't reached a consensus on the ideal body fat percentage, they do agree on a range. For men, depending upon age, the range is between 12 and 22%, and for women 16 to 30%. These figures need to be interpreted with caution, and you shouldn't become obsessed with the numbers. The numbers can fluctuate depending upon the test used, the tester, and the testee. In addition, this is just one assessment tool, and it should not be given inordinate emphasis. However, if you are at the high end of the scale, then you should be concerned.

DETERMINING YOUR
BODY FAT PERCENTAGE

There are several different ways to determine your body fat percentage. None are consistent and you might score 24% percent using one method and 29% percent using another. You might even get widely varying results using the same test, depending upon the skill of the tester, your physical condition, and the condition of the equipment.

Tests Requiring Equipment & Skilled Testers:

WATER WEIGHING
This test requires you to blow ALL of your air out of your lungs and stay underwater for five seconds. If you have air trapped in your lungs, the results make you appear fatter than you are. While this is a cumbersome, somewhat costly test, it still is the most accurate.

BIO-ELECTRICAL IMPEDANCE
This is a simple, non-invasive test that involves attaching electrodes on your feet and hand and measuring the speed of the electrical signal passing through your body. Muscle is 70% water and fat is 5-13% water, and since electricity passes more quickly through water, the slower the signal, the more fat you have. This test has limitations. For example, if you are extremely fat or lean, there can be a large margin of error. Dehydration can skew the results because the less water your body has, the slower the signal. Thus, you'll appear to have more fat than you actually have.

CALIPERS

This is the most common test and also the most widely varying test. The tester takes some tongs that look like giant tweezers and measures the thickness of your body fat at three to seven body locations. The skin-folds are measured in millimeters and are plugged into a formula to determine your body fat percentage. The tester should pinch each site 2-3 times.

There are limitations to this test, too. The tester might not pinch exactly the same spot or pull out the same amount of fat from the bone. He might pinch too hard and yank some of your muscle along with your fat. To preclude some of these errors, have the same tester each time and be tested at the start of your workout. (After exercise, blood travels to your skin to cool you down, thus causing your skin to swell and you will test fatter than you are.)

Where can you have these tests performed?

Most university physical education or health departments, health clubs, and hospital clinics can do these tests. While there will probably be a charge, it should be minimal.

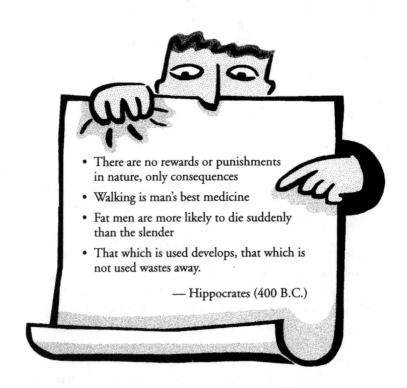

- There are no rewards or punishments in nature, only consequences
- Walking is man's best medicine
- Fat men are more likely to die suddenly than the slender
- That which is used develops, that which is not used wastes away.

— Hippocrates (400 B.C.)

Body Composition Tests That Can Be Done at Home With Little Equipment

PINCH TEST TO MEASURE BODY FAT
This simple test can be done in the privacy of your home, and in a matter of seconds, you can accurately measure your body-fat percentage.

MEN: Pinch a fold of soft tissue on the abdomen and measure it's width. A reading of 3/4" represents a body fat percentage of 13-18%. A measurement of 1" means a percent of 18-22%.

WOMEN: Use soft tissue on back of upper arm. A measurement of 3/4" equals 18-23% body fat, 1" equals 24-28%.

BOTTOM LINE: If you can pinch an inch or less, you've passed the pinch test. CONGRATULATIONS!

TANITA BIO-ELECTRICAL IMPEDANCE ANALYSIS
Tanita produces several scales in the $50 - $90 range that use the bio-electrical impedance analysis (BIA) to determine body fat percentage. Based on your height, weight, sex, and the speed at which a safe, low level electrical signal passes through the muscle and fat, you get an accurate body fat reading. The process takes a few seconds. These scales are available at major retail stores. The Scale Plus Body Fat Monitor stores data for four people. www.tanita.com.

BODY MASS INDEX (BMI)
The Body Mass Index (BMI) is one of the easiest and cheapest test. It can be done at home and all you need to know is your height and weight in pounds. The average BMI for Americans is 26.3. In terms of RealAge the ideal BMI is 23 or less. If you have a BMI of 23 or less you can have a RealAge as much as eight years younger than if you had the national average of 26.3.

CAUTION: The BMI can be misleading. It has the same limitations as the scale. The BMI fails to distinguish between fat and muscle. It can overestimate the fat in people who are very muscular and underestimate body fat in people who have lost muscle mass, such as the elderly. The BMI should be viewed as one of many measures of health. Other important functions are cardiovascular-fitness level and muscle strength.

FIND YOUR BODY MASS INDEX (BMI)

Weight in pounds (weight without clothes)

5' 1"	100	106	111	116	122	127	132	137	143	148	153	158	185	211
5' 2"	104	109	115	120	126	132	136	142	147	153	158	164	191	218
5' 3"	107	113	118	124	130	135	141	146	152	158	163	169	197	225
5' 4"	110	116	122	128	134	140	145	151	157	163	169	174	204	232
5' 5"	114	120	126	132	138	144	150	156	162	168	174	180	210	240
5' 6"	118	124	130	136	142	148	155	161	167	173	179	186	216	247
5' 7"	121	127	134	140	146	153	159	166	172	178	185	191	223	255
5' 8"	125	131	138	144	151	158	164	171	177	184	190	197	230	262
5' 9"	132	135	142	149	155	162	169	176	182	189	196	203	236	270
5' 10"	136	139	146	153	160	167	174	181	188	195	202	207	243	278
5' 11"	140	143	150	157	165	172	179	186	193	200	208	215	250	286
6' 0"	140	147	154	162	169	177	184	191	199	206	213	221	258	294
6' 1"	144	151	159	166	174	182	189	197	204	212	219	227	265	302
6' 2"	148	155	163	171	179	186	194	202	210	218	225	233	272	311
BMI (%)	19	20	21	22	23	24	25	26*	27	28	29	30	35	40

Table Courtesy of American Institute for Cancer Research

BMI FORMULA   *EXAMPLE: 6', 191 LBS. = 26% BMI

1. Multiply your weight (lbs.) x 705

2. Divide result by your height (in inches)

3. Divide again by your height (in inches)

4. Answer: _____

INTERPRETING YOUR BMI

- A BMI between 18.5 and 25 carries little health risk. Try to keep your weight within this healthy BMI range.

- A BMI of 25-30 is considered overweight and carries some increased health risk.

- A BMI over 30 is defined as obese and poses the greatest risk to your health.

- A BMI greater than 40 requires medical attention.

ARE YOU AN APPLE OR A PEAR?
WAIST - HIP RATIO TEST

Another method used to determine your BMI is called the waist to hip ratio.

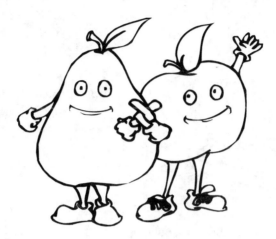

- Standing relaxed, measure your waist and hips (at their widest points) with a tape measure.

- Divide your waist measurement by your hip measurement. (For a man with a 36" waist and 38" hips, the result is .95. For a woman with a 32" waist and 40" hips, the result is .80)

- Men may have to lose weight if their ratio is 1.0 or higher; women, if their ratio is .80 or higher.

The waist-hip ratio test is based on research indicating that where you are genetically programmed to store fat may be more important than how much fat you have. Men and women who carry excess fat primarily around their midsections (apples) have been known to have a higher risk of diabetes, heart disease, stroke, and certain types of cancers than people who carry it primarily on their hips and thighs (pears).

- My Waist measurement is:_____
- My Hip Measurement is:_____
- My Waist to Hip Ratio is:_____ (Waist/Hips. Example: 36/38 = .95)

WHAT ARE YOU ... APPLE OR PEAR?

DO I NEED TO LOSE WEIGHT?
... PUTTING IT ALL TOGETHER

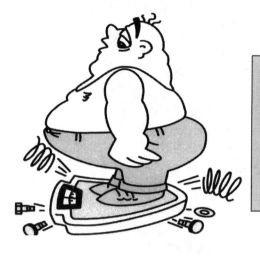

> **DEFINITION OF DRESSING ROOM PHOBIA:**
>
> *A fear of trying on clothes in dressing rooms, commonly caused by ineffective fad diets, non-existent exercise routines and the rollercoaster of yo-yo dieting.*

1. Do I have a health condition that would benefit from weight loss?   Yes   No

2. Am I an apple or pear?   Apple   Pear

3. Will weight gain affect my quality of life, now or later?   Yes   No

4. Is my BMI outside the acceptable range?   Yes   No

5. Do I have any unhealthy habits, i.e. smoking, excess alcohol, poor food choices?   Yes   No

WHAT WORKS

If you answered more of the left column, it is an indication that you need to lose weight. Here's what you can do:

- Make a commitment.
- Set realistic goals for weight loss and fitness.
- Learn to enjoy healthful food, not pills or fad diets. This is for life!
- Exercise daily.
- Adopt a healthy lifestyle (no smoking, moderate or no alcohol, good food choices).

CHAPTER THREE:
EXERCISE GUIDELINES

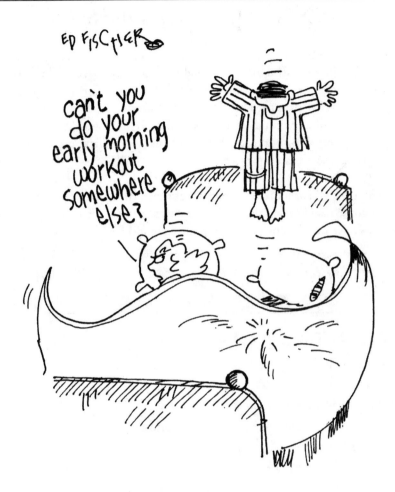

Energize With Exercise!

Spring to action! Start the day with a peppy workout that boosts the body's energy by twenty-five percent. Get off the bus or park the car farther from your destination and walk.

(Reprinted with permission from Dr. Jeff Haebig, Wellness Quest©)

The only way to get rid of fat permanently is to increase physical activity and decrease the fat in your diet!

EXERCISE GUIDELINES

If you're going to be successful in losing weight and getting fit, you MUST commit yourself to a planned program of exercise and stick with it. This means scheduling 30 + minutes a day, five days per week for physical activity. This schedule of exercise should be thought of as essential as a proper diet. We must give exercise the same priority as we give brushing our teeth on a daily basis. We can have our teeth replaced a lot easier and cheaper than our heart!

Activity can play a very important role in weight loss. Although people who do not engage in exercise may lose weight by cutting down their caloric intake, people who are regularly active find it much easier to reduce fat and KEEP IT OFF.

> *"The best nursing home insurance you can have is physical fitness."*
> *— Steven Blair, Ph.D., Aerobic Institute*

25 REASONS TO EXERCISE

1. Reduces body fat.
2. Live longer and BETTER.
3. Reduces chances of heart attack.
4. Builds and maintains bone density (prevent osteoporosis).
5. Increases heart/lung efficiency.
6. Lowers resting heart rate.
7. Lowers blood pressure.
8. Improves skin elasticity and tone.
9. Reduces stress, tension, and depression.
10. Sleep better.
11. Raises the HDL (good) cholesterol and lowers the LDL (bad) cholesterol.
12. Increases muscle strength and endurance.
13. Enhances sexual desire, performance and satisfaction.
14. Improves flexibility.
15. Recover from operation/illness quicker.
16. Improves digestion/elimination.
17. Slows the aging process.

18. Reduces back pain.
19. Improves performance in work and play.
20. Look and feel better.
21. Reduces appetite.
22. Increases metabolic rate.
23. Burns fat calories.
24. Lowers blood sugars and decrease risk of diabetes.
25. Reduces medical and healthcare expenses.
    AND MANY, MANY MORE.

Lack of exercise has been cited as the most important cause of "creeping" obesity in modern, mechanized societies. Few occupations now require vigorous physical activity. By switching from a typewriter to a computer keyboard, a secretary gains 6-7 lbs. of fat per year. The average American spends 4-6 hours per day watching television. In the early years of television, one would have made 12-15 trips from the couch to the TV to adjust the volume, change channels, etc. Now we sit in the chair and not only operate the TV but answer the phone with our portable model.

ANY CONNECTION?

1996 Study: Over 60% of population get no regular physical activity
2002 Study: Over 61% of population are overweight

Using the TV remote control can add 7 lbs. of fat to our bodies. Most people no longer walk to the store, school or work. We even ride in an electric cart when we play golf. Although we have more time available for recreation, many people do not use leisure time for activities that give them exercise.

21st Century Couch Potato:
- Full time job, sits at desk all day
- 3 nights a week at meetings – sits
- Runs errands – in car
- Plays games – poker, bridge – sits
- Mows lawn – riding lawnmower
- You are a couch potato if the longest time you spend in continuous full-time movement is less than 15 minutes, twice a week.

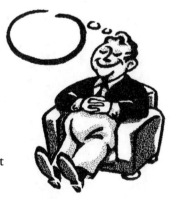

SURGEON GENERAL'S REPORT ON EXERCISE

On July 11, 1996, the Surgeon General issued a 13-word warning:

"The Surgeon General warns that physical inactivity may be hazardous to your health."

This was the third report issued by the Surgeon General. In 1964, the first report alerted the nation to the hazards of smoking. Over the years, it has done much to change the social norm concerning smoking. In 1988 the Surgeon General issued a report on nutrition and health, which focused attention on the need for sound nutrition. The main message of the Physical Activity and Health report in 1996 was that Americans can substantially improve their health and quality of life by including MODERATE amounts of physical ACTIVITY in their DAILY lives. The greatest gains for personal health come when people move from a sedentary to an active lifestyle.

Unfortunately, the old 80/20 Rule that applies to so many areas of our life also applies to fitness and health. Only 20% of the population are active enough to get the physical and mental benefits of regular activity.

The most important goal in the eyes of public health officials is to get people who are totally sedentary (20% again) to do something. The next most important goal is to get the 54% who do very little to do a little more.

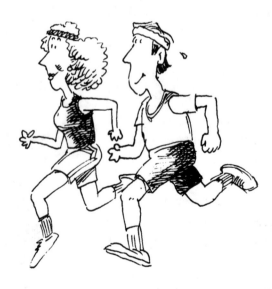

Following are the major findings of the Surgeon General's Report:

- Every U.S. adult should accumulate 30 minutes or more of moderate intensity physical activity on most, preferably all, days of the week.
- Physical activity need not be strenuous to achieve health benefits.
- Physical activity need not be continuous to achieve health benefits.
- Greater health benefits can be achieved by increasing the amount of physical activity.
- Activity includes household chores such as washing windows, cleaning floors, etc.

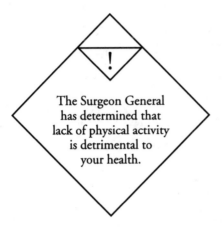

The Surgeon General has determined that lack of physical activity is detrimental to your health.

President's Council on Physical Fitness and Sports
2010 Adult Fitness Objectives

An increased percentage of the American population will:

- **ENGAGE** in moderate physical activity for at least 30 minutes, five days per week. **GOAL:** Increase from 15% to 30%
- **ENGAGE** in vigorous physical activity three or more days per week for 20 or more minutes per occasion. **GOAL:** Increase from 23% to 30%
- **PERFORM** strength and endurance activities two or more days per week. **GOAL:** Increase from 18% to 30%
- **PERFORM** physical activities that enhance and maintain flexibility at least once every two weeks. **GOAL:** Increase from 30% to 43%

"GET AMERICA MOVING" – PRESIDENT'S FITNESS CHALLENGE. Free program for tracking activities and earning badges. (www.presidentschallenge.org) 800-258-8146

For information on the President's Council on Physical Fitness and Sports call: 202-690-9000

EXAMPLES OF MODERATE
AMOUNTS OF ACTIVITY

- Washing and waxing a car for 45-60 minutes
- Washing windows or floors for 45-60 minutes
- Playing volleyball for 45 minutes
- Playing touch football for 30-45 minutes
- Gardening for 30-45 minutes
- Wheeling self in wheelchair for 30-40 minutes
- Walking 1 3/4 miles in 35 minutes (20 min./mile)
- Basketball (shooting baskets) for 30 minutes
- Bicycling 5 miles in 30 minutes
- Dancing fast (social) for 30 minutes
- Pushing a stroller 1 1/2 miles in 30 minutes
- Raking leaves for 30 minutes
- Walking 2 miles in 30 minutes (15 min./mile)
- Water aerobics for 30 minutes
- Swimming laps for 20 minutes
- Wheelchair basketball for 20 minutes
- Basketball (playing a game) for 15-20 minutes
- Bicycling 4 miles in 15 minutes
- Jumping rope for 15 minutes
- Running 1 1/2 miles in 15 minutes (10 min./mile)
- Shoveling snow for 15 minutes
- Stair walking for 15 minutes

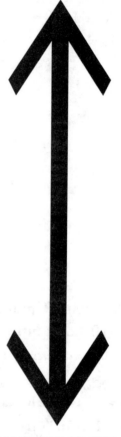

LESS VIGOROUS,
MORE TIME

MORE VIGOROUS,
LESS TIME

EXERCISE DOESN'T HAVE TO BE REGIMENTED.
THE MAIN THING IS TO MOVE!

A moderate amount of physical activity is roughly equivalent to physical activity that uses approximately 150 calories of energy per day, or 1,000 calories per week. Some activities can be performed at various intensities; the suggested duration should correspond to expected intensity of effort.

ABOUT EXERCISE INTENSITY AND MONITORING YOUR EXERCISE PACE

Heart rate at rest and during exercise is an important measure of fitness. In order to improve your aerobic fitness, it is necessary to get your heart beating faster at a steady and sustained rate for a minimum of 15 to 20 minutes (30-45 minutes as you become better conditioned).

The two most common methods for monitoring your intensity are Target Heart Rate and Perceived Level of Exertion.

Target Heart Rate

About 80% of the population can make good use of pulse monitoring during and after exercise to judge the intensity of their exercise. The two most common locations to take exercise pulse are the inside of the wrist (brachial artery) or the side of the neck just below the jaw (carotid artery). For both locations, apply slight pressure using the index and middle finger.

If you monitor your heart rate, here are some terms you should be familiar with:

RESTING HEART RATE (RHR) is the number of times your heart beats per minute when you first wake up – before you sit up. The average American has a RHR of 72, but exercise will lower this number significantly, indicating your heart has become more efficient and requires less work to do its job.

AMBIENT HEART RATE (AHR) is the number of beats per minute your heart beats when you are wide awake and in a sedentary and upright position. Most people use the Resting Heart Rate when they mean the Ambient Heart Rate. The AHR can be taken any time after rising.

MAXIMUM HEART RATE (MHR) is the number of times your heart pumps when it's working at 100% capacity. This number generally decreases as you age. The formula for determining MHR is 220 minus your age. Example: (220-50 (age) = 170 MHR). **NEVER EXERCISE AT THIS RATE!**

TARGET HEART RATE (THR) is the number of beats per minute your heart should beat to provide effective aerobic training for your age and fitness level.

FITNESS FORMULA • F. I. T. T. S.

Frequency	= How often?	5-6 times per week
Intensity	= How hard?	60-85% MHR
Time	= How long?	30+ minutes
Type	= Activity?	Walking
Social	= Exercising with a Buddy	

Determine your target heart rate from the chart on the next page. Check your pulse at the beginning of your exercise routine to determine your starting level. An easy method for taking your pulse during exercise is to take it for 6 seconds and add a zero (multiply by 10) to figure out your 60 second pulse. Check your THR 5 - 10 minutes into your exercise. If you're below the THR, exercise a little faster; if you're above the THR, slow down. Try to keep your heart rate within the target range for at least 20 minutes.

TOTAL TRAINING SESSION

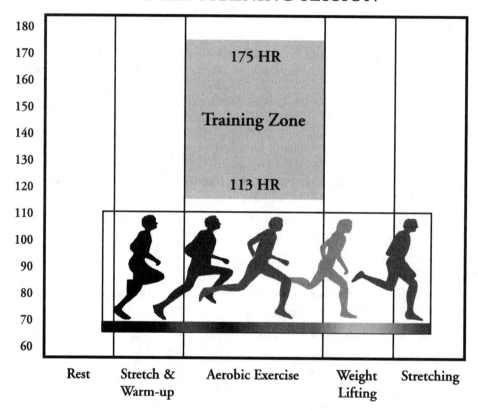

HEART RATE TRAINING ZONES

- MAXIMUM Target heart rate for a 45 year old exercising at 85% MHR would be 175. (220 - 45 x 85%)

- MINIMUM Target heart rate would be 113. (220 - 45 x 60%)

FINDING YOUR TARGET HEART RATE (THR)

(220 - Age x _____% = THR)

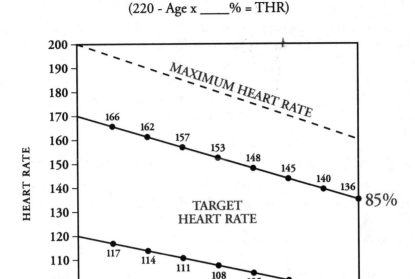

REMEMBER: If you have not exercised in a long time and are overweight, DO NOT EXCEED THE 60% LEVEL FOR THE FIRST 4 WEEKS.

After you have been exercising for some time, you will sense what it feels like to have your heart rate within the target zone. Use the following table to chart your progress.

Resting Heart Rate & Target Heart Rate

	BEGINNING	AT 5 WEEKS	AT 10 WEEKS
WRITE DATES HERE			
MY RESTING HEART RATE			
MY TARGET HEART RATE			

CAUTION: If you are on medication, i.e. heart, blood pressure, and other related medication, be aware that the above heart rates may not apply as your heart rate will be limited at rest and exertion. If this applies to you, check with your doctor, and you may want to use the Perceived Exertion Scale described next.

PERCEIVED LEVEL OF EXERTION

Until recently, monitoring your pulse and keeping it in a certain range based on your age was the most common way to determine if you were exercising "hard" enough. However, we now know that monitoring the pulse is not always effective because it is difficult to get an accurate measure since so many factors can alter your pulse. Experts feel that for 10-20 % of the population, the target heart rate does not apply. Studies have also shown that in water exercise the target heart rate is lowered by 10-15 %.

Today most exercise specialists believe the effective way to monitor your exercise is what Covert Bailey calls the talk test. Exercise guru Bailey describes it this way. "Say you are jogging with a friend. Is he able to talk, but you are not? Each of you should be able to talk a little bit, but neither of you should be able to sing an aria." In scientific terms, the talk test is called the Borg Rating of Perceived Exertion. It is a scientifically reliable and valid indicator of physical exertion.

Perceived exertion refers to the physical strain individuals believe they are experiencing while exercising. A rating of 4 corresponds to approximately 60% of a person's maximum oxygen capacity (VO2 max.) A rating of 6 corresponds to approximately 80 - 85%. Exercising at levels 3 - 4 is adequate for burning fat, but for fitness training a level of 4 - 6 is recommended.

PERCEIVED LEVELS OF EXERTION

Perceived Exertion (PE)	How Hard?	Breathing	Can You Talk?	% Max. HR
1	Very Easy	Normal	Until Someone Interrupts	35
2	Easy	Still Normal	"As I was saying…"	45
3	Light, but starting to feel like exercise	Comfortable	No problem yet	55
4	Somewhat hard	Noticeably Deeper	Possible, but no soliloquies	65
5	Hard	Deep but steady	Just name, rank, serial number	75
6	Between hard & very hard	Deep & getting faster	Name only	85
7	Very hard	Deep and fast	Initials only	90
8	Very, very hard	Very deep, very fast	Maybe a grunt	95
9	So hard you can only do it for a few seconds	Panting	A gasp	97.5
10	Maximum effort	Can't breathe	Can't even gasp	100%

EXERCISING AT 100% MAY BE DANGEROUS

HEART MONITORS

Wearing a heart rate monitor has become as commonplace as putting on a wristwatch. Thanks to modern technology and a drop in price, people are finding that monitors can help them lose weight, feel better, decrease stress, and reduce the risk of exercise-related injuries.

A heart rate monitor can let exercisers know if they're exercising appropriately. You're probably saying, "Why can't I just take my pulse in my neck or wrist as you've outlined previously?" According to studies performed by Dr. James Rippe and published in the New England Journal of Medicine, taking a pulse during exercise is intermittent and may be inaccurate by as many as plus or minus 15 beats per minute. Also, other muscle movements and heavy breathing can make a pulse difficult to find and count. Finally, if exercisers stop or slow their activities to count, it's not really an accurate measurement.

Some people are unable to get results from a heart monitor. Prior to my bypass heart surgery in 1999, I was unable to get a reading from a heart monitor. However, the rhythmic problem was corrected during the surgery and as a result, I now wear a monitor during my treadmill and aerobic workouts. By using this simple device, I am able to keep my heart rate within my target range with no problem.

Recently, during a 5 km race-walk, I wanted to keep my exercise heart rate within the 120 beats per minute (75% MHR) to 136 bpm (85%) range. By wearing the heart monitor, I could keep a check on my rate. During the race, I found myself unknowingly being over 150 bmp (95%) on several occasions, and it was easy to ease up without stopping to take my pulse.

There are several different methods of measurement. The heart rate monitors that provide continuous readings use the same technology that is found in hospital cardiac labs. The monitor has two components: the transmitter worn around the chest that picks up electrical from the heart and the receiver, which picks the signal from the transmitter and displays it in watch-like fashion.

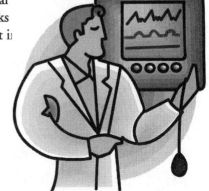

Heart Monitors are available in four categories. Entry-level ($60), Mid-level ($90-$120), advanced ($120+) and competitive ($200+). One popular brand is Polar (800-227-1314. www.polarusa.com).

EXERCISE JOURNAL

For the week of _____

DAY	ACTIVITY	MINUTES	DISTANCE	COMMENTS
SUNDAY				
MONDAY				
TUESDAY				
WEDNESDAY				
THURSDAY				
FRIDAY				
SATURDAY				

COMMENTS

Maybe you're a runner. Maybe you're the fastest since Secretariat. But if running is the extent of your exercise program, you're probably NOT totally physically fit. While your cardiovascular fitness may be second to none, and you have thighs to rival Barry Sanders, what about your upper body strength, your flexibility, and your tendency for overuse injuries? Runners tend to have problems in these areas.

By mixing up your activities at least twice a week, you can reach fitness levels you've never seen before and avoid overuse injuries and boredom.

FITNESS SMORGASBORD

Instead of spending 30-60 minutes on the same machine, why not do an exercise smorgasbord?

- SKI MACHINE
- STEPPER
- TREADMILL
- ROWER
- EXERCISE BIKE
- ELLIPTICAL TRAINER

Select three fitness machines and do 10 minutes on each.

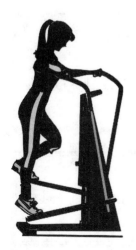 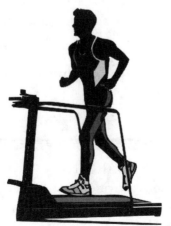 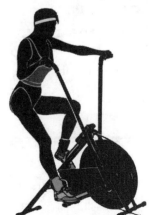

DAY	ACTIVITY	BEGINNER	INTERMEDIATE	ADVANCED
		Cal/30 min. Easy pace (PE – 3)*	Cal/30 min. Moderate pace (PE – 4-5)*	Cal/30 min. Hard pace (PE – 6)*
MON	SWIM	240 calories	380 calories	440 calories
TUE	W .L.	200	320	400
WED	BICYCLE	160	320	400
THUR	ROWING	140	280	340
FRI	W. L.	200	320	400
SAT	WALK (60 min) RUN (30 min)	240	380	440
SUN	REST			
	TOTAL CAL.	1180	2000	2420

Based on 175 lb. person.   *See chart on "Perceived Level of Exertion."

WARNING:

These are strenuous activities. Start at the beginner level
and gradually increase the intensity.

15 EXERCISE GUIDELINES

1. SET REASONABLE GOALS:
Goals should be achievable. In the enthusiasm of the moment, many people set goals that are too high. It's good to dream, but do so with some realism.

My exercise goals are:_____

_____

_____

2. START SLOWLY:
You didn't get out of shape overnight, and you won't get in shape overnight.

3. STICK WITH IT:
Don't get discouraged and quit if you don't see quick results or if you miss one or two days.

4. FIND A PARTNER:
If you can find someone who has a similar goal and is at your same physical level, you'll find exercising together makes the time pass more quickly.

My support group includes:_____

_____

_____

5. SET A REGULAR TIME FOR EXERCISE:
There is no right time to exercise. The best time for you is the time that you will "just do it." Whatever your preference, establish a definite time and stick with it.

6. MONITOR YOUR HEART RATE:
Don't exceed your exercise heart rate or perceived level of exertion.

7. DON'T OVERDO:

Your body is your best indicator for this. Your body will tell you when it is fatigued and worn down. When it does, slow down. Many exercisers adopt a hard-easy training program. One day will be a hard workout and the next day, an easier one so that the body has time to recuperate.

8. DON'T IGNORE PAIN:

The old saying "No pain, no gain" is a falsehood. Exercise should not be painful. If it is, you're doing something wrong. Exercise does involve effort. Sweat is okay; pain is not! If you experience pain, reduce your activity level. If the pain does not go away, see your doctor.

9. KEEP AN EXERCISE AND DIET JOURNAL:

Studies have shown that recording your exercise and eating goals, as well as charting your progress, is a proven way to stay focused and motivated. A "Dietminder Personal Food and Fitness Journal" can help you keep your New Year's resolutions. (www.memoryminder.com)

10. CROSS TRAIN:

This means to vary your activities. Instead of walking or swimming every day, you substitute weights, cycling, or tennis. Many athletic injuries are the result of overuse by repeating the same movement patterns. With cross training you never do one activity long enough to get into trouble.

11. DON'T DO DANGEROUS EXERCISES:

Certain exercises such as straight leg sit-ups and full squats are not safe for your back.

12. INCREASE LIFESTYLE ACTIVITY:

Use stairways instead of elevators at work, walk during coffee breaks, park in the farthest spot from your office or the mall, get rid of the remote control on your TV. Remember extra activity burns additional calories.

I can increase my lifestyle activity by_____

_____

_____

13. AVOID GETTING SIDETRACKED BY LIFE:

There will be days you have to miss your exercise program. Don't let a temporary lapse turn into a collapse. If you have a goal of lifetime fitness, one or two days is in significant in the master plan of life. Your goal is to exercise for LIFE!

14. DRESS FOR COMFORT AND SAFETY:

Wearing worn out or improperly sized shoes will lead to injuries. If you exercise at night wear reflective clothing. Dress in layers. As your exercise warms your body, you can remove layers and put them back on as you cool down.

15. LISTEN TO YOUR BODY:

Probably the most important rule is: when your body says, "I'm working too hard," slow down.

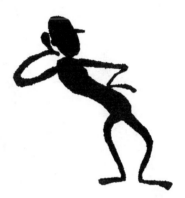

SPINNING: A TOTAL BODY WORKOUT

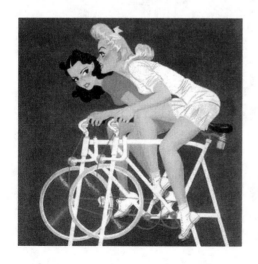

Spinning is the latest fitness craze. Using a stationary bike that has a 40 lb. flywheel spinning provides a full body workout. The ride is usually done in a group and starts out with a warm-up, followed by a simulated ride on a flat road, seated climb, standing climb, sprints on a flat road, and jumps on a hill. This ride takes you through various heart-rate zones. Each rider adjusts his/her own resistance and pedal speed. The workout is usually done with music.

EXERCISE PRESCRIPTION
FOR TOTAL FITNESS

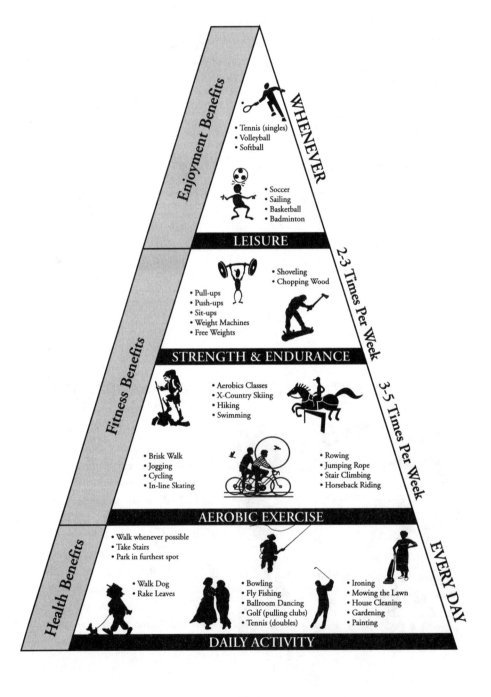

Enjoyment Benefits

WHENEVER

- Tennis (singles)
- Volleyball
- Softball

- Soccer
- Sailing
- Basketball
- Badminton

LEISURE

2-3 Times Per Week

- Shoveling
- Chopping Wood

- Pull-ups
- Push-ups
- Sit-ups
- Weight Machines
- Free Weights

STRENGTH & ENDURANCE

Fitness Benefits

3-5 Times Per Week

- Aerobics Classes
- X-Country Skiing
- Hiking
- Swimming

- Brisk Walk
- Jogging
- Cycling
- In-line Skating

- Rowing
- Jumping Rope
- Stair Climbing
- Horseback Riding

AEROBIC EXERCISE

- Walk whenever possible
- Take Stairs
- Park in furthest spot

EVERY DAY

Health Benefits

- Walk Dog
- Rake Leaves

- Bowling
- Fly Fishing
- Ballroom Dancing
- Golf (pulling clubs)
- Tennis (doubles)

- Ironing
- Mowing the Lawn
- House Cleaning
- Gardening
- Painting

DAILY ACTIVITY

AEROBIC TRAINING CHART

Try to get some kind of physical activity at least 5 days each week.

	WEEK 1							5 Days/Week	
	Sun	Mon	Tues	Wed	Thurs	Fri	Sat	Yes	No
Time									
Activity									
	WEEK 2								
Time									
Activity									
	WEEK 3								
Time									
Activity									
	WEEK 4								
Time									
Activity									
	WEEK 5								
Time									
Activity									
	WEEK 6								
Time									
Activity									
	WEEK 7								
Time									
Activity									
	WEEK 8								
Time									
Activity									
	WEEK 9								
Time									
Activity									
	WEEK 10								
Time									
Activity									
TOTAL DAYS EXERCISED:									

Use the following codes to record your daily activity.

Some activities will be more vigorous than others. Certain activities develop strength and flexibility, while others develop aerobic endurance.

Code	Activity
BM	Badminton
BB	Basketball
CA	Calisthenics
CS	X-Country Skiing
C	Cycling
DN	Dance
DN/A	Dance/Aerobic
JO/R	Jogging/Running
MA	Martial Arts
RHS	Racquetball/Handball
RJ	Rope Jumping (Individual)
R	Running
SW/L	Swimming/Laps
WA	Water Aerobics
T	Tennis
V	Volleyball
WA	Walking
WT	Weight Training

Business travel provides a wealth of excuses not to exercise. We sleep through the hotel alarm. We opt to go out and wine and dine with our colleagues instead of going to the gym. We use the lack of time excuse; we can't block off a 60 minute segment of time. Instead of doing 2-3 brisk 10 minute segments, we do nothing. We use the excuse that we don't have access to the exercise machines that we use at home and ON and ON and ON.

David Chamberlain, former CEO of Shakley, USA says, "I have a theory on life that we always find the time to do the things we like to do and never have the time to do the things we don't like to do. There isn't a Hyatt or Marriott that doesn't have a place to go and get a pretty good workout."

Regular exercise is especially vital for business travelers. Not only does it recharge your batteries, it fills your body with much needed oxygen, increases your productivity, and reduces stress.

12 Ways to Stay in Shape While Traveling

1. On-site health clubs. Most hotels cater to fitness conscious travelers. Check your hotel out BEFORE signing in.
2. Gym in a suitcase. See below. Always have a bag packed and ready to go.
3. Local gyms and spas. Most have guest drop-in rates.
4. Go for a walk. Most hotels have maps of areas that are safe for walking or running – if not, just walk the halls and stairways.
5. Stair climbing. Climb 2 flights of stairs (no faster that 2 steps per second) and rest by taking a one minute walk on level ground.
6. Walk to your meetings.
7. Use the hotel's pool and do water aerobics or lap swimming.
8. Eat right. Even though you're away from home, don't forget to "eat right."
9. Drink lots of water.
10. Always pack your fitness gear.
11. Do a morning stretch.
12. JUST DO IT!

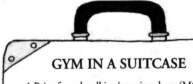

GYM IN A SUITCASE

1 Pair of good walking/running shoes (MOST IMPORTANT) • 1 pair of good athletic socks
Walkman • 1 cassette or CD of relaxation music
Set of exercise bands • Jump Rope
Water inflatable dumbbells (2, 5, 10 lb sizes)
Tubing • Pair of exercise shorts and shirt
Bathing suit • 1-2 Aerobic video tapes
Jogging suit • Good pedometer

10 INEXPENSIVE FITNESS TOOLS
THAT WORK

Americans are always looking for new and better (easier) ways to get fit. If you've ever (and who hasn't) been lured by the promises of the TV pitchmen, you know that these "get fit" gadgets rarely deliver. Remember the "Butt Blaster," "Ab Blaster," "Cardio and Aerobic Riders," "Solo Flex" and on and on?

Here are 10 fitness tools that deliver what they claim to (listed alphabetically):

Digi Walker Kit:
($25-30, depending on model). The Digi Walker is covered in the Walking Chapter. You can purchase a pedometer in the store that gives you steps and distance, but for the same price you can get the Kit from Rob Sweetgall that will give you programs and knowledge to help you reach your goal of 10,000 steps per day.

Exercise Journals:
($10). These are covered in the Walking Chapter.

Exerstriders:
($75). Look like modified ski poles or walking sticks and come in varying lengths. Studies show that these poles utilize all of your body's major muscles and that you consume 20-50% more oxygen than a regular walking workout.

Heart Rate Monitors:
($50 and up). These were covered extensively in the section on heart rate monitoring. There are many brands. Decide ahead of time what features you need and don't buy a lot of frills that you won't be using.

Jump Ropes:
($3-10). They can be carried in your suitcase, used in your home fitness circuit, or at work during a break. Be sure to get the right length, with comfortable handles and a sturdy rope. A source for ropes, bands, balls, mats, and stretch cords is SPRI at 1-800-222-7774.

Resistance Bands:

($5-15). These bands are ideal to take in your suitcase. They effectively strengthen any body part from feet to shoulders. They come in different sizes and widths. They come in sets with varying elasticity and an illustrated exercise book.

Stability Balls:

($20-30). These inflatable balls were originally used to aid children with cerebral palsy, stroke victims and back injuries. The balls are now used in fitness to promote flexibility, balance, strength and coordination. These are discussed in the Flexibility Chapter.

Stretch Cords:

($10). Cords are different than bands. Cords improve flexibility and are ideal to use for cool down stretches or to assist in the rehabilitation of muscle injuries. They can also be used in yoga to enhance the effects of certain poses.

The Stick:

($25-40, depending on the model). The Stick is discussed in the chapters on stretching and stress. There are many models designed to reach all parts of the body. My wife owns four Sticks and won't leave home without one in her suitcase.

Water Shoes and Web Gloves:

($15-60). These are a necessity if you do water aerobics on a regular basis. The shoes maintain a grip on the pool floors that sometimes tend to be slippery, and the gloves enable more water to be pulled, providing greater resistance.

---

10 TIPS FOR STAYING MOTIVATED:

1. Vary your routine or change your scenery
2. Try something entirely new
3. Find a workout buddy
4. Set a new goal
5. Treat yourself to a workout gadget or accessory
6. Keep an exercise log to track your progress
7. Don't berate yourself if you miss a workout
8. Reward yourself
9. Focus on how good exercise makes you look and feel
10. If all else fails, take a break from exercise

— *American Council on Exercise (ACE)*

CHAPTER FOUR:
STRETCHING GUIDELINES

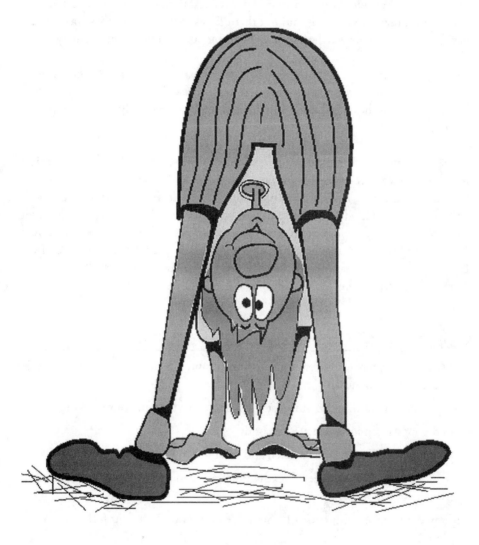

*"To restore life to your life,
to defeat aging,
to regain the youth you still possess,
get your body in motion."*

— Aristotle

STRETCHING GUIDELINES

Warming up, cooling down, and stretching are not the most exciting topics, but as you get older, they become more and more important. Think of your muscles as rubber bands; warm them up properly and put them to rest properly, and they stay soft and flexible. But put them away hot, they will become stiff and lose their elasticity.

Flexibility is so important that it should have a separate place in your fitness plan. Try to spend 15-30 minutes at least 3 times a week doing a stretching routine, starting with your head and neck muscles and working gradually down the body to the toes.

Stretching is the key to maintaining flexibility, posture, muscle balance, and injury prevention. Please re-read the previous sentence and, consider its significance. Flexibility means that we can stand up straight, bend down without pain, and walk with fluid strides. Good posture means that your head, neck, shoulders, back, thigh, and hip muscles are in alignment, and chances are you will avoid back discomfort. Muscle imbalance occurs when one muscle (for example the quadriceps or front thigh muscle) becomes stronger than the rear or hamstring muscle. This leads to altered muscle movements, clumsiness, and even pulled muscles.

Stretching Rules

- Always warm up before stretching. For maximum benefits, stretch after both the warm up and cool down.
- Stretch all of your muscles, not just the ones you've used in your workout.
- Hold each stretch for at least 15 seconds
- Don't bounce. Ease into the stretch and hold it.
- Breathe normally. Take deep breaths inhaling through your nose and exhaling through your mouth.
- If you experience pain, back off. Stretch to a point where you feel tension and hold it.

There are some basic stretches that you can do before or after exercise. Some people stretch before they work out to lengthen the muscles for use. Others prefer to stretch after the workout, when the muscle is warm because that is when it is more flexible. Whenever you choose to stretch, don't bounce or do ballistic movements. Instead, move slowly into position, then hold the stretch for 10-15 seconds. According to some exercise physiologists, stretching should receive 10% of your workout time.

WARMING UP/COOLING DOWN

Many people believe that stretching and warm up are the same. While you can incorporate stretches in the warm up process, they are different. A good 15-20 minute stretching program should be done 2-3 times a week independent of your aerobic workout. Warming up before your aerobic exercise is a good idea. It prepares the heart and other muscles for the activity ahead. Warm up for 5-10 minutes at the beginning of each workout by doing a slower, gentler version of your aerobic activity. For example, walk slowly before you fitness walk. By emphasizing the same muscles you plan to use in your main activity, you'll warm them up gradually. If you want to do a few stretches in your warm up, include them at the end of the warm up.

> *People who are out of shape need to warm up the longest. Their bodies aren't accustomed to movement, whereas the more fit you are, the more your body remembers what it's supposed to do and warms up quicker.*

The length of your warm up depends upon several factors: your physical condition, the length and intensity of your upcoming workout, and any physical problems you may have. People who are out of shape need to warm up the longest. Their bodies aren't accustomed to movement, whereas the more fit you are, the more your body remembers what it's supposed to do and warms up quicker. Also, the longer and harder you plan to work out, the longer you need to warm up. If you have any muscle soreness or weakness, it is best to warm the muscle thoroughly before starting any workout.

Cooling down is just as important as warming up.

Cooling down returns the muscles to their pre-activity level and it helps to reduce the after exercise soreness by eliminating any lactic acid that may have accumulated in the muscles during the exercise period. If you are exercising hard and don't cool down, your blood pressure can plummet quickly. You might feel weak and dizzy, get sore muscles, or even pass out. Many exercise authorities feel that the cool down is more important than the warm up. **If you are only going to do one, choose the cool down.**

Remember not to count the warm up and cool down periods as part of your 30 minute workout.

20 SECOND TOTAL BODY STRETCH

If you have to sit for long periods try this total body stretch. It will help combat the aches and pains that sneak up on the body.

Door Stretch:

1. Find a narrow doorway. Lay your forearms up against each side of the doorway, with one foot behind the other and begin to lean forward. As you lean forward, your shoulders will be pulled back.

2. This will stretch your chest muscles as well as the shoulder muscles. You can control the force of the stretch by moving your front leg farther forward.

3. By turning toward one side, you will stretch the muscles above the rib cage. Maintain this stretch for 20 seconds.

4. Then put the other foot forward and repeat.

> *Stretching is the key to maintaining flexibility, posture, muscle balance, and injury prevention.*

FACTORS THAT AFFECT FLEXIBILITY

- **AGE** — People lose about 40% of their flexibility between the ages of 20 and 70.
- **INACTIVITY** — Causes tissue in the joints to shorten.
- **GENDER** — Women tend to be more flexible than men.
- **MUSCLE DENSITY** — Thicker people have broader muscle fiber which is harder to stretch.
- **ATHLETIC EXPOSURE** — If you are exposed to flexible sports (gymnastics, cheerleading, etc.) early in life, you can carry that flexibility longer in life.
- **INJURY** — Whether it's because of damage to the tissue, scarring, or lack of use, injury can affect flexibility.

STRETCHES FOR WARM-UP & COOL-DOWN

(SEE DIAGRAMS ON PAGE 57)

These stretches should be done after a 5-10 minute warm-up, and/or at the end of the workout. To warm-up you may do a slow run or walk. These stretches are designed to be done in the upright position and the 10 stretches can be done in 5 minutes or less. There are literally hundreds of stretches and you are encouraged to develop your own set of stretches which can be done 2-3 times a week, separate from your workout. The following stretches are not designed to take the place of those stretches; but are designed to stretch the muscles used in your aerobic workout. Notice that they start from the top of the body (shoulders) and work down to the bottom (ankles). Each stretch (excepting stretches 4, 9 & 10) should be done for 20 seconds.

1. ***Behind the Back Shoulder Stretch:*** Start in a standing position. With your hands behind your back, join the fingers of both hands together. Straighten both arms and raise your hands as high as comfortable behind your back. Hold the position.

2. ***Above the Head Shoulder Stretch:*** Start in a standing position. Place your right arm over your head with your elbow bent. Grasp your right elbow with your left hand and gently pull your right elbow behind your head. Hold this position. Repeat this exercise with the left arm.

3. ***Side Stretch:*** Place both arms straight above your head and lean to the left. Stretch all of the muscles along the right side of your body. Hold this position. Repeat leaning to the right.

4. ***Inner Thigh and Groin Stretch:*** Gradually spread your legs until you feel a stretch on the inside of your thighs and groin. Use hands for balance. Hold an easy stretch for 30 seconds. Be careful of over-stretching, particularly at the beginning.

5. ***Hamstring Stretch:*** Place your foot on an object (railing or fence) at or below hip level. Don't get your foot higher than what is comfortable. Lean forward from your hips without rounding your upper back. Try to keep your back straight. Slightly bend the knee of your supporting leg to increase the intensity of the stretch. Repeat with the opposite leg.

6. ***Quadriceps Stretch:*** Bend the knee and gently lift the heel to buttock level. Use the opposite hand to hold the ankle and pull upward. With your free hand, hold on to a stationary object for balance. Repeat with opposite leg. **(People with knee problems should use caution or skip this stretch.)**

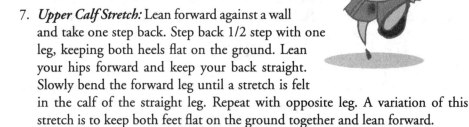

7. ***Upper Calf Stretch:*** Lean forward against a wall and take one step back. Step back 1/2 step with one leg, keeping both heels flat on the ground. Lean your hips forward and keep your back straight. Slowly bend the forward leg until a stretch is felt in the calf of the straight leg. Repeat with opposite leg. A variation of this stretch is to keep both feet flat on the ground together and lean forward.

8. ***Lower Calf Stretch:*** Do the same exercise as #7, but this time bend the rear leg slightly. Repeat with opposite leg.

9. ***Ankle and Achilles Stretch:*** This is often referred to as the heel raise. Stand with feet apart, shoulder width. Raise up slowly on the toes and briefly hold. Do 25 times.

10. ***Shin Stretch:*** This is the reverse of the heel raise. Slowly lean back on the heels, bringing toes up to point to the sky (ceiling) and briefly hold. Do 25 times.

TIP: The above two (ankle and shin) stretches are great ones to do while you are pumping gasoline into your car. It certainly is better than standing there watching your money disappear. Of course the people around you might wonder what you are doing, but it's great for starting conversations.

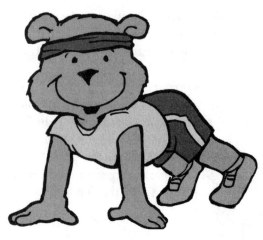

TEN WARM-UP STRETCH EXAMPLES

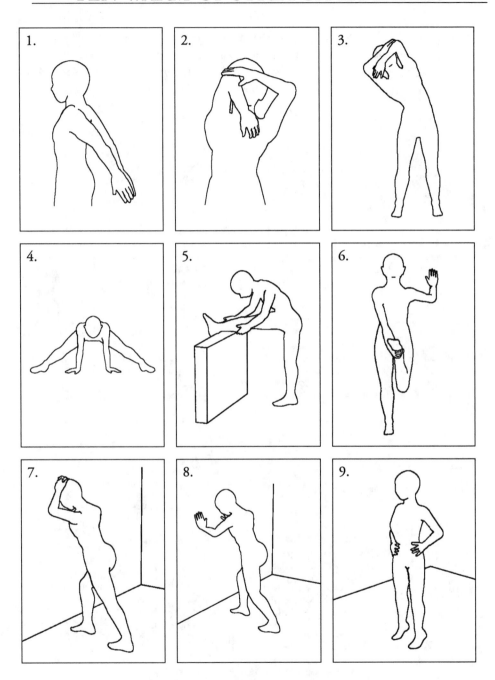

10. Reverse of number 9. Point toes up toward the ceiling and balance on heels.

10 Great At-Your-Desk Exercises: *If you're one of the millions of Americans who spend most of their work day behind a desk, you know it helps to take an exercise break to ease muscle tension and to get the blood circulation. Here are 10 great at-your-desk exercises to use when you don't have the time to take a walk:*

① **Knee Kiss.** Pull one leg to your chest, grasp with both hands, and hold for a count of five. Repeat with opposite leg.

② **Windmill.** Place your feet apart on the floor. Bend over and touch your right hand to your left foot, with your left arm extended up. Repeat with opposite arm.

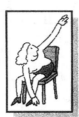

③ **Back Relaxer.** Bend down between your knees as far as you can. Return to upright position, straighten, and relax.

④ **Pectoral Stretch.** Grasp your hands behind your neck and press your elbows back as far as you can. Return to starting position, then drop your arms and relax. Repeat.

⑤ **Middle-Upper Back Stretch.** Raise your right arm and grasp it below the elbow with your left hand. Gently pull your right elbow toward your left shoulder as you feel the stretch. Hold for five seconds. Do both sides.

* If your desk chair has wheels, use caution!

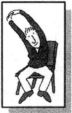

⑥ **Side Stretch.** Interlace your fingers. Lift your arms over your head, keeping your elbows straight. Press your arms backward as far as you can. Then slowly lean to the left, and then to the right, until you can feel stretching.

⑦ **Fingers.** With your palms down, spread your fingers apart as far as you can. Hold for the count of five. Relax. Repeat.

⑧ **Shoulder Roll.** Slowly roll your shoulders forward five times in a circular motion, using your full range of motion. Then roll your shoulders backward five times with the same circular motion.

⑨ **Neck.** Let your head drop slowly to the left, then to the right. Slowly drop your chin to your chest, and then raise your chin as high as you can. Turn your head to the left, return it to the normal position, and then turn it to the right.

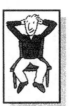

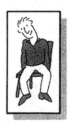

⑩ **Quadriceps.** Bring your legs straight out in front of your body, and then hold them in that position for five seconds. Make sure you are sitting up straight. Relax. Repeat.

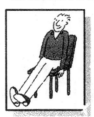

Reprinted with permission: Hope Publications, Kalamazoo, MI 616-343-0770

EXERCISE BALLS

Recently, the exercise ball was named as one of the top 10 most effective fitness gadgets invented during the nineties. It is a fun, safe, and highly effective way to exercise. It can be used for strength building, stretching and flexibility, aerobic workouts, and injury rehabilitation.

Some uses are:

- Use when stretching, strength building and working on abs. Most exercise physiologists feel it is much superior to the traditional crunches. In one report, a fitness editor sat on a ball at her desk for 6 weeks and developed abs that are the envy of the office without doing a single crunch.
- Use as a chair replacement. This would be an excellent chair to use while "surfing" the net.
- Balls can be used in rehabilitating injured knees, back, neck, and shoulders.
- Ball dancing while watching TV will stimulate your metabolism and bounce away a few calories.

These are just a few uses for a very inexpensive fitness prop.

BALL BUYING TIP

Using the wrong size can reduce the safety and effectiveness of your workout.

YOUR HEIGHT	BALL SIZE
4'8"- 5'3"	55 centimeters
5'3"- 6'0"	65 centimeters
6'0"- 6'7"	75 centimeters

NEW KIND OF OFFICE CHAIR

Want tight abs without doing crunches? Try sitting on a Ball Chair!

Those 25" inflatable exercise balls used for strength building, stretching and aerobic workouts can also be used as a desk chair! The ball makes it tough to slouch and encourages a slight bouncing movement that keeps leg and back muscles busy and eases stress. TRY IT!

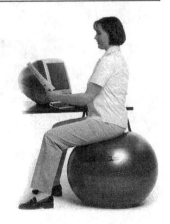

MUSCLE SORENESS?

"THE STICK" makes your muscles feel better in seconds. This portable, self massaging device is simple, effective and inexpensive. It rapidly increases blood circulation and locates, and releases trigger points (knots in your muscles). A complete body rollout takes less than 10 minutes.

The award winning STICK has been clinically proven by thousands of physicians and therapists since 1989. You can experience the exhilaration of taking care of your personal well-being, and you can partner up with others to share this amazing device. All it takes is 30 seconds per muscle group. In summary, the STICK is guaranteed to make the muscles feel better, work harder, last longer, and recover faster. Prices range from $26 - $40.

Personal Testimony

Sharon, my wife, suffers from fibromyalgia. This is characterized by sore muscles and ligaments throughout the body. She has been using the STICK since 1996 and will not leave home for more than a day without it! I take my stick to the club and use it after a workout. Between my wife and I, we must have 6 different STICKS, each designed for different purposes. The STICK is being used by many professional athletes.

For more information on THE STICK, go to www.dumpyourplump.com and click on "health links" or call: Rainbow Wellness at 269-925-3524.

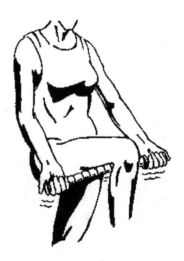

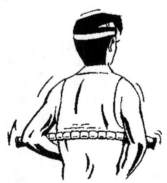

A PRIOR PHYSICAL PROGRAM
PREVENTS (BACK) PAIN

The 5 P's (Prior Planning Prevents Poor Performance) was one of the mantras I used when I supervised the Army medical clinics at Camp Grayling and Camp Ripley. I always tried to do a meeting outline prior to conducting a meeting. Likewise, I would never discuss a problem without first having thought it through.

In prevention of back pain, a prior physical program (aerobics, strengthening, and stretching) will eliminate or greatly lessen the severity of back pain. It is an accepted fact that 80% of us will at some time in our lives experience back pain. I venture to say that in actuality the figure is probably closer to 100%.

Our back works nonstop to support us in walking, sitting, standing, playing, and even lying down. Given such a heavy task, it's no wonder back pain affects most of us sooner or later. Fortunately, there are ways to "save" our back.

It would be presumptuous on my part to try to tell you in a couple of pages how to "cure" back pain when there are so many causes. Countless books have been written on the subject. There is no such thing as "one cure fits all." Studies have shown that back problems are caused by a variety of reasons, i.e. genetics, obesity, poor posture, turning the "wrong" way, improper lifting, fatigue, stress, etc. If you have the following symptoms, you are advised to seek medical assistance. Start with your family physician, chiropractor, internist, or osteopathic doctor who can either treat you or refer you to the appropriate specialists, i.e. orthopedic or neurosurgeon, acupuncturist, or physical therapist, depending upon the severity.

> ## SEEK MEDICAL HELP
> ## IF YOUR PAIN
> *... is unremitting, regardless of your posture.*
> *... is the result of a traumatic accident.*
> *... involves bowel or bladder problems.*
> *... follows an illness or fever.*
> *... is severe and extends below the knee.*
> *... includes numbness, weakness,*
> *or tingling below the knee.*

Personally, I have had much success with chiropractic treatment, physical therapy, massage, and acupuncture when it comes to back pain. My rule of thumb with these alternative forms of medicine is that you should begin to feel relief within a few visits. If you don't, you should look elsewhere. If you can avoid back surgery, it is to your benefit as, unfortunately, back surgery is not successful in many situations. I would rather start with the least invasive treatment, instead of having surgery as my first option.

Twelve years ago I was advised by a neurosurgeon that I needed immediate surgery for my back pain. I had a second opinion (which I always advise), and I was advised to begin a preventive exercise program and delay the surgery, which I've been able to do.

While there are numerous causes for back pain, most causes trace back to a sedentary lifestyle. People with low levels of physical fitness tend to have weaker abdominal and back extensor muscles which promote the majority of support for the back. Therefore, we need to take care of our back, so our back can take care of us.

SELF HELP FOR BACK STRAIN

1. Apply a cold compress for 15 minutes, four times a day for the first 48 hours.

2. Take an over the counter anti-inflammatory pain reliever (aspirin or ibuprofen) to reduce the swelling.

3. Take it easy; but more than a couple of days in bed can make it worse.

4. Return to activities slowly.

BACK SAVING EXERCISES

Warning: Do not attempt these exercises without medical approval if you are currently experiencing back discomfort.

1. **KNEE/LEG RAISE (Hip Flexor)**
   Lie on your back with both legs straight (knees can be bent), feet flat on the floor and arms at your sides. Do a pelvic tilt (explained in #3A) and hold.

   1A: Grasp one thigh behind your knee and pull it toward your chest and hold for 3-5 seconds.

   1B: Then, slowly straighten the knee and raise your leg as high as possible without pain. When your leg is raised, pull it closer to you and hold for 3-5 seconds. Repeat with the other leg.

   Do 5-10 repetitions per leg.

2. CAT-CAMEL (Warm-up)

This stretch warms up the spine by slowly flexing and extending your spine, similar to what a cat does when first getting out of bed.

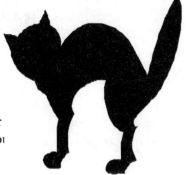

2A: CAT: Get down on hands and knees with hands shoulder width apart. Slowly lower your between your arms as you push up as high as you with your back.

2B: CAMEL: When you reach the top of the movement slowly lower your back as you extend your neck forward and up. Arch your lower back by pushing your navel toward the floor.

That's one repetition. Do 5-10 repetitions.

3. CRUNCH (Abdominal)

3A: Lie on your back with both knees bent and feet flat on the floor. Cross your arms across your chest. Do a pelvic tilt (rotate your pelvis so your lower back comes in contact with the floor. Tighten your lower abdominal muscles.)

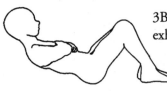

3B: Keep your lower back in contact with the floor, exhale, and slowly raise your shoulder blades off the floor, then lower them, inhaling as you return to the starting position. Keeping your eyes on the ceiling, try not to bend your neck forward.

Hold for 5 seconds. Repeat 5-10 times.

4. SPINAL FLEXION (Lumbar & Lower Back)

Bend forward slowly while sitting. Reach as far as you can until you experience mild discomfort. Hold this position for 15 seconds. Repeat 3-5 times.

5. WALL SLIDE (Abdominal and Thigh)

5A: Stand with your back against the wall, feet shoulder width and heels 12-18" from the wall. Exhale and do pelvic tilt (see 3A above) so the lower back comes in contact with the wall.

5B: Bend your knees while sliding your back down the wall. Bend your knees as far as comfortable. DO NOT EVER BEND THE KNEES MORE THAN 90 DEGREES! Hold the bottom position for 10-20 seconds.

Repeat 5-10 times.

BACK EXERCISES

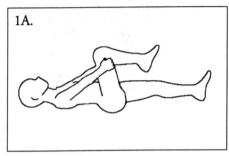

1A.

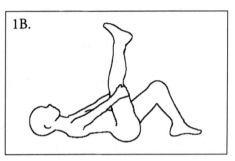

1B.

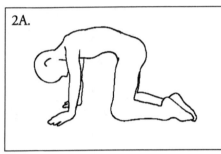

2A.

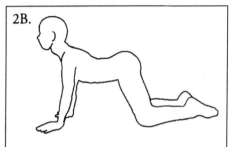

2B.

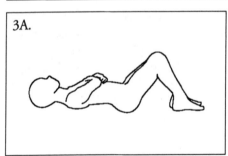

3A.

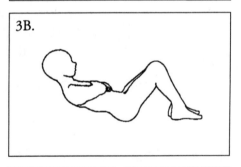

3B.

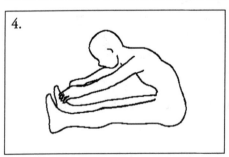

4.

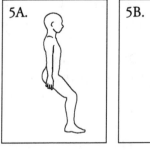

5A.

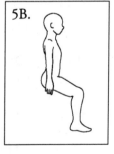

5B.

1A.	Knee Raise	2B.	Camel	4.	Spinal Flexion
1B.	Leg Raise	3A.	Crunch	5A.	Wall Slide
2A.	Cat	3B.	Crunch	5B.	Wall Slide

Take care of your back so it can take care of you!

- **SHRINK YOUR ABDOMEN.** The more it protrudes, the more it strains your back. I have a 20 lb. "fat belly" that I have people wear so they can see for themselves what effect extra weight has on the body.

- **GET REGULAR AEROBIC EXERCISE.** Aerobic (non-stop) exercise can increase the flow of oxygen to the back muscles.

- **DO A WEIGHT LIFTING WORKOUT.** Strength training 2-3 times a week is VERY important. Strengthening the four major muscles (abs, quads, and hams) stabilizes the spine.

- **SIT PROPERLY.** Your lower back should rest against the seat cushion. No slouching.

- **TAKE SITTING BREAKS.** Try to stand up every 30 minutes and walk around.

- **GET PLENTY OF SLEEP.** The body recuperates during rest. Fatigue hinders good posture.

- **SHOES.** Don't skimp on your shoes. Wear cushiony, supportive shoes. Use orthodics if necessary. Avoid high heels.

- **STRETCH.** When sitting or standing for long periods, do gentle stretches. When driving take stretch breaks every 1-2 hours.

IT'S TIME TO GET STARTED

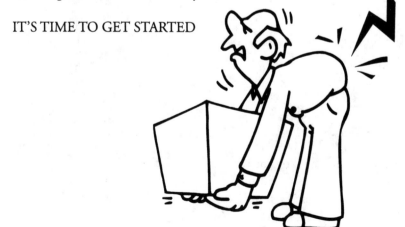

SUN SALUTATION

The Sun Salutation is a yoga exercise that incorporates poses that flow from one to the next. It is a great exercise to do in the morning to get the blood flowing and stretch all your muscles. NOTE: This exercise can also be good for the back. Do movements slowly. Hold each pose for 1 -2 seconds. Ease up if you feel pain!

1. Stand with feet together and arms by sides. Inhale as you reach arms up overhead until palms touch. Look at hands. Keep shoulders down (MOUNTAIN POSE).

2. Exhale to FORWARD BEND; knees bent and hands touching floor, with chest resting next to thighs.

3. Inhale as you bend left knee and extend right leg back to a lunge. Place hands on both sides of your front foot (LOW LUNGE).

4. Exhale and bring left leg back in line with right, keeping head, torso and legs in one line for PLANK POSE. (Similar to the push-up starting position.)

5. Lower legs and torso to floor, so you're lying flat on your stomach. Hands are under your chest. Then slowly raise head, neck, and shoulders up in a curve without arching your back. (COBRA POSE.)

6. Push onto hands and feet, lifting hips to the sky to form an upside-down V. This is known as the DOWNWARD-FACING DOG.

7. Return to COBRA POSE.

8. Bring right foot forward and return to lunge, keeping left leg straight behind you (LOW LUNGE).

9. Bring left foot up to meet right and return to FORWARD BEND.

10. Inhale; sweep your arms out and up.

11. Exhale and come back into the first standing posture (MOUNTAIN POSE). Hold and bring arms down to side.

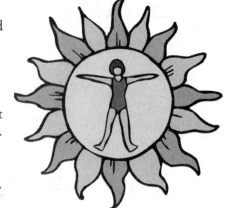

12. This is one set. Repeat entire sequence. Try for 5-10 sets.

CHAPTER FIVE:
STRENGTH TRAINING

USE IT OR LOSE IT!

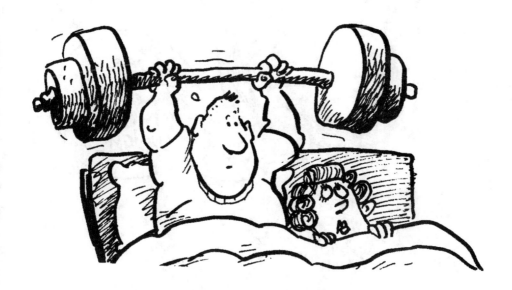

*"Weight lifting can do as much for the inside of the body
as it does for the outside. If you use weights in a moderate way,
you can gain a wide range of health benefits."*

— Kerry Stewart, Ed.D
John Hopkins School of Medicine

DEVELOP OVERALL STRENGTH

As we get older, strength training becomes so important. Beginning at age 25, we lose 5-10% of our muscular strength every ten years of our lives. Nothing is more true when it comes to, "You use it or you lose it" than when it is applied to our muscles. Unless, we get into a strength program to reverse this loss, we can expect a future of diminished quality of life.

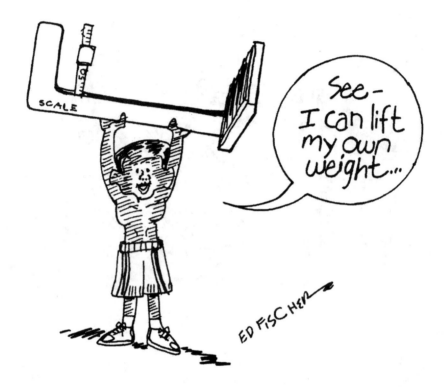

(Reprinted with permission from Dr. Jeff Haebig, Wellness Quest©)

GAIN MUSCLE – LOSE WEIGHT

"Every pound of new muscle requires 50 calories a day at rest for tissue maintenance. When you replace 5 pounds of fat with 10 pounds of muscle, your weight remains the same, but you can expect to expend 2500 or more additional calories each day at rest. That translates into 2 lbs. per month!"

— Wayne Wescott, YMCA Fitness Research Director

In <u>Biomarkers</u>, Dr. William Evans documents how weight training can positively affect 10 vital biological markers: (Evans)

Biomarker 1	Your Muscle Mass
Biomarker 2	Your Muscle Strength
Biomarker 3	Your Basal Metabolic Rate (BMR)
Biomarker 4	Your Body Fat Percentage
Biomarker 5	Your Aerobic Capacity
Biomarker 6	Your Body's Blood-Sugar Tolerance
Biomarker 7	Your Cholesterol/HDL Ratio
Biomarker 8	Your Blood Pressure
Biomarker 9	Your Bone Density (Osteoporosis)
Biomarker 10	Your Body's Ability to Regulate Internal Temperature

Undoubtedly, this is a pretty impressive list which adds importance to weight training. Is 20 minutes, three times a week too much to ask for when all of the above benefits are considered? For additional information the purchase of Biomarkers is recommended.

Dr. Evans was one of the researchers that conducted the landmark study on aging and strength training in which a group of 90 year old men and women increased their strength by an average of 174% after just eight weeks of three days a week on weight machines. Several were able to move out of their wheel chairs because of their increased strength. The oldest individual was 96 years old!

After the age of 25, the average male loses 8 lbs. of muscle mass every ten years and the average female loses 5 lbs. until menopause and then 10 lbs. every ten years. This becomes very critical when the person reaches 60-70 years old as they have lost the muscle strength needed to perform basic walking and lifting tasks.

> *The more muscle you have, the more calories you can consume without gaining weight.*

Many people, especially women, shy away from weight training because they're afraid of developing big muscles and looking muscle bound. Ninety nine percent of the adults can't look like Arnold Schwarzenegger or Cory Everson (champion body builders) regardless how much they try. As a matter of fact, overweight people will actually be smaller. There will be a decrease in body fat with an increase in lean body mass (muscle), and we all know that muscle takes up less room than fat. However, more importantly, the more muscle you have the more calories you can consume without gaining weight. Since muscles use more calories than fat (96% of our calories are consumed by our muscles), it stands to reason that the person who has more muscle mass can eat more food without gaining weight. Basal metabolic rate (the number of calories your body consumes at rest) is determined largely by lean body tissue or muscle. The less muscle you have, the lower your metabolism-and the easier it is to gain weight. Compare it to the gasoline car engine. The larger the horsepower (muscle) of the engine (body), the more gas (calories) the car (body) consumes. We should all be trying to maintain a diesel engine in a streamlined chassis. Someone once said, "muscles are workhorses, fat is a storehouse. Your body needs more workhorses and fewer storehouses."

Turn Back the Clock

Studies have shown increases of 4-7 lbs. of muscle tissue after four months to one year of weight training. This corresponds to an increase of 6-12% in metabolism. According to Dr. Wayne Wescott, raising our metabolism rate by 7% reverses 14 years of the aging process.

As a general rule, women genetically have less muscle and more body fat. Therefore, "pumping iron" helps to counteract the body's natural tendency to replace muscle with flab. At 20, the average woman has 23% body fat; the average man 18%. At 35, those numbers are up to 30% and 25% respectively. By the time 60 rolls around, fat has claimed 44% of a woman's body and 38% of a man's.

Surprisingly, aerobic activity alone won't stop this muscle-to-fat progression. Studies have shown that endurance-sport exercisers lose large amounts of muscle mass and strength by their 60's, even when they're aerobically fit. Lifelong weight lifters, on the other hand, can maintain muscle strength into their 70's. When Danish researchers looked at 70-year-old men who swam, ran or lifted weights regularly, they found that while the swimmers and runners had lost as much muscle as sedentary 70-year-old controls, the weight lifters had muscle strength and composition comparable to 28-year-olds.

In the mid 1990's, Jeff Everson, Editor of Muscle and Fitness Magazine, said: "No one will ever convince me that weight training is not the best thing for middle aged and older individuals. Within 10 years, every physician will prescribe weight training for nursing home patients, just as they prescribe walking now." Unfortunately, his prediction has not come true.

After the age of 25, the average male loses 8 lbs. of muscle mass every ten years. This loss of strength can be prevented with a minimum of 60-90 minutes of strength training per week.

This loss of strength can be prevented with a minimum of 60-90 minutes of strength training per week. There are 6 basic tasks that we want to be able to do until the last day of our lives: dress ourselves, bathe ourselves, take care of our toilet needs, walk a moderate distance, be able to play with our grandkids, and be able to travel. All of these depend upon a minimal strength level that we can maintain with a modest strength program.

In the mid 1980's, for the college weight-lifting class I taught, I began using a circuit program (explained later in this chapter) which combined lifting with aerobic activity. Prior to this time, the students were on a 3 set, 10 repetition lifting program which was the standard weight lifting protocol. The students were always given a pre and post test (something everyone should do). At the end of the semester, we found that the difference in strength level between those who did three sets of each lift, versus those who did the circuit was not significantly different. However, what was statistically different was that the cardiovascular level of the students who did the circuit program was significantly higher. These results corresponded to the results of studies conducted by leading exercise physiologists.

To digress a moment, there are basically five components to a physically fit person: flexibility, muscle strength, muscle endurance, aerobic capacity, and weight management. Many runners, swimmers, and aerobic dancers are fine in the weight management and aerobic capacity, but fail miserably in the muscle strength, muscle endurance and flexibility areas. As Dr. Evans has so ably pointed out in his Biomarkers book; that, as we get into our 60's, muscle strength and flexibility play increasingly important roles.

Therefore, if a person says they only have 30 minutes a day, five days a week to exercise, it is important that at least two of those days and preferably three (nonconsecutive days) are spent on the circuit program. The circuit can be done at home or at the local gym. More and more commercial fitness clubs have recently included the circuit program in their offerings.

LIFTING WEIGHTS WILL:

- BOOST METABOLISM by increasing your body's muscle mass.
- CHANGE THE SHAPE OF YOUR BODY. For example, it can sculpt shoulders, raise buttocks, lift the chest.
- STRENGTHEN MUSCLES, JOINTS AND LIGAMENTS, minimizing the risk of injury.
- INCREASE BONE DENSITY, a strong factor in preventing osteoporosis.

"This may come as a shock to 'cardio-fanatics' but strength training is the single most important and effective exercise to help boost metabolism."
— *Kathy Smith, Fitness Guru*

LIFTING WEIGHTS WILL NOT:

- WORK YOUR HEART AND LUNGS. You still need a separate cardiovascular workout, such as walking!
- MELT POUNDS IMMEDIATELY, since muscle weighs more than fat. But in the long run, it helps you lose.
- INCREASE FLEXIBILITY. Be sure to stretch your muscles every day and especially after every workout
- BREAK THE BANK. Weights don't cost a lot; some weight exercises (push-ups, crunches) don't require any.
- BULK UP YOUR MUSCLES. A bodybuilder's physique is achieved through intense training and, sometimes, genetic predisposition.

71

SIT-UPS VS. CRUNCHES

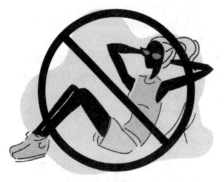

Those of us from the old school grew up with the idea drummed into our heads that if you wanted flatter "abs," you had to do sit ups. The Army Physical Fitness Test (APFT) consisted of a timed run, push-ups and sit-ups. All of the services had similar fitness tests. However, in the late 1980's the Navy got rid of the sit-ups and the Marine Corp did so in 1998. Both services cited concerns about lower back injuries caused by the rocking motion produced by sit-ups. The Air Force recently added crunches to its fitness assessment, thus the Army is the lone service that requires the traditional sit-up. To make matters worse, the Army still requires the sit-up be performed with the hands locked behind the neck, instead of resting on the chest.

According to Major Richard Baxter, physical therapist at West Point's Department of Physical Therapy, "Sit-ups cause a tremendous amount of compression on the discs in the lumbar spine and create tremendous shear force on the lumbar spine as well. They can cause low-back strains and injuries to the discs. Someone who does sit-ups for years and years can end up with degenerative disc or spinal problems and arthritis."

I don't know if I can blame my spinal problems on sit-ups or not. When I was in high school, I established the school record for sit-ups — something like 900; and unfortunately, I did them for many years. In my role as the fitness officer in my military assignments, I can recall some serious injuries as a result of improperly performed sit-ups.

Fortunately, most people are now doing crunches which put less stress on the lower back. You assume the same position as the sit-up, except when you come up, you only curl your upper body to the point where the shoulder blade leaves the ground. That way, the lumbar spine - the lower back - stay flat on the ground and is not being pulled up into a vertical position, so you avoid the stresses on the lower back and neck.

FLATTER ABS.

The American Council on Exercise (ACE) sponsored a study of the "best" and "worst" abdominal exercises for achieving stomach-flattening results. They evaluated 13 of the most common abdominal exercises, some involving equipment, some not. The top three most effective were **BICYCLE MANEUVERS, CAPTAIN'S CHAIR,** and **CRUNCHES ON AN EXERCISE BALL.** To view these exercises, go to: www.acefitness.org.

BASIC PRINCIPLES
FOR STRENGTH TRAINING

- **NUMBER OF EXERCISES:** You should do at least 8-12 strength exercises that address all major muscle groups. (See muscle chart)

- **FREQUENCY:** Two to three nonconsecutive times per week. In other words, M, W, F or T, F etc.

- **SETS:** One is sufficient.

- **RESISTANCE:** 70-80% of maximum resistance (1RM). One way is to experiment until you have found a weight that you can lift 8 times, but not 10 times.

- **NUMBER OF REPETITIONS:** 8-12 for upper body-When 12 can be lifted without too much effort, increase to the next weight level (the increase should not be more than 10%). 12-17 for lower body-When 17 is reached, increase to next level (no more than 10% increase). This is called "progressive resistance."

- **LIFTING SPEED:** Slow to moderate, two seconds for the lifting and four seconds for the lowering.

- **ORDER OF EXERCISES:** Usually you want to do upper body, lower body, upper body, lower body, etc. This gives the exercised muscle a chance to recover.

- **RANGE OF MOTION:** Full range when possible.

FOUR R'S OF STRENGTH TRAINING

RESISTANCE: (overload) To get stronger, a muscle must be exposed to demands that it has not yet experienced. Increases must be small. (5 - 10%)

REPETITIONS: Must be done in deliberate, controlled fashion (no jerking) and through the greatest range of motion. While numbers can vary, the general rule is 12 reps. When this can be done correctly, the resistance is increased (progressive resistance).

RECOVERY: A muscle doesn't get stronger during a workout, but AFTER a workout. Allow at least 48 hours for maximum growth. Example: Lift - Monday - Wednesday - Friday.

RECORDS: Very critical. Records document your history and identify plateaus. Progress indicates that the first three R's of strength training (resistance, repetitions, and recovery) have been applied correctly.

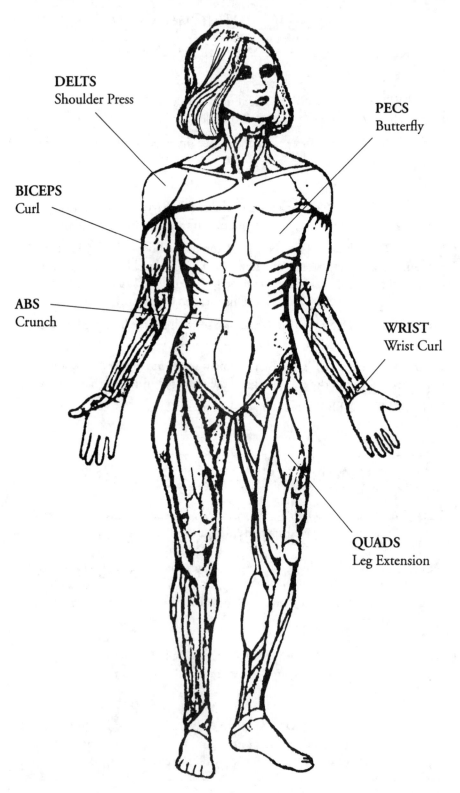

DELTS
Shoulder Press

PECS
Butterfly

BICEPS
Curl

ABS
Crunch

WRIST
Wrist Curl

QUADS
Leg Extension

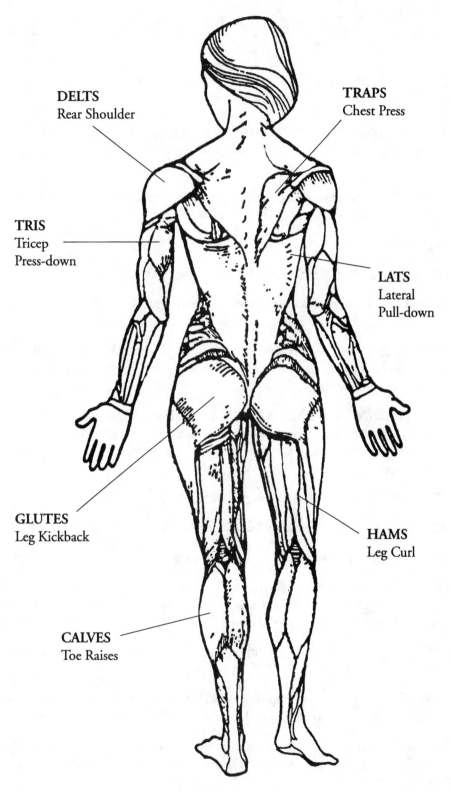

DELTS
Rear Shoulder

TRAPS
Chest Press

TRIS
Tricep
Press-down

LATS
Lateral
Pull-down

GLUTES
Leg Kickback

HAMS
Leg Curl

CALVES
Toe Raises

WEIGHT TRAINING JARGON

Here are a few buzzwords and their definitions so that you can hold your own during conversations in the gym or over the water cooler.

BENCH PRESS: This is the best exercise for the upper body. The lifter takes a supine position on the bench and moves the weight from chest level to a straight arm position.

CURLS: From a standing position start with your arms extended to the floor, palms up grip. Raise the bar to near chin level, then lower the bar back to the starting position.

CUTS: Muscular development reflected by separations between muscle groups.

DUMBBELL: Short barbells from 8" to 20" long. Very versatile.

ISOMETRIC: The static contraction of a muscle group in which the joint angle and muscle length remain constant, i.e. pushing the palms together and holding.

NEGATIVE EXERCISE: Exercises that limit the muscle's movement while increasing the muscle's length, i.e. slowly lowering the weight in the bench press under complete control.

OVERLOADING OR PROGRESSIVE RESISTANCE: When you are able to do the desired number of reps correctly, then you increase the poundage or resistance by approximately 5% and use that weight for workouts. Most efficient way to increase strength.

PYRAMIDING: Increasing the weight after each set.

REPS: Repetitions. A rep occurs when you perform a complete cycle of movements.

SET: Completion of desired reps. For basic muscular strength 10 reps is the usual goal.

SPLITS: An advanced program in which a person lifts six days a week, but never two days in a row on the same muscle groups, i.e. Mon/Wed/Fri-glutes, quads, hams, calfs, abs and Tues/Thur/Sat-back, chest, shoulder, triceps and biceps. Sunday is a rest day.

STICKING POINT: Lifting point at which maximum effort is required to complete the move.

SUPER SETS: Working two opposing muscles with little or no rest between the sets, i.e. leg extension (quads) and leg curls (hamstrings) or biceps and triceps curls.

TEN REPS MAX (RM): This is the maximum number of reps of an exercise that can be done with a set poundage. The person is unable to do more than 10 Reps at this weight.

CIRCUIT TRAINING
AT A COMMERCIAL CLUB

Depending upon the facilities this can be done a multitude of ways. You can use a Walkman tape player so that it won't be disruptive. The problem with doing it at the club is that unless you pick an off time, you will have to stop and wait for people to finish their routine. Some clubs designate periods where they have machines set aside for people using a circuit program and then it becomes very easy to work out.

How to start out:: Start lifting light weights (something you can do 15-20 times) and do each weight and aerobic exercise for 60 seconds followed by a 15 second move to the next exercise. As you gain strength and endurance, gradually increase the weight. This is NOT an easy workout!

Here is one possible workout: (See "Circuit Training Diary")

STRENGTH:	AEROBIC:
1. Bench press	2. Bike
3. Leg extension	4. Ski machine
5. Lateral Pull down	6. Stepper
7. Leg Curl	8. Treadmill
9. Shoulder Press	10. Jump rope
11. Abdominal Curl	12. Rowing Machine
13. Back Bend	14. Bike
15. Lateral Raise	16. Ski
17. Butterfly	18. Stepper
19. Bicep Curl	20. Treadmill
21. Tricep Press-down	22. Jump Rope
23. Toe Raise	24. Rowing
25. Heel Raise	

NOTE: If you desire to do only a strength workout, do only the weight training strength exercises. If you desire only an aerobic workout, do the aerobic activities.

CIRCUIT TRAINING DIARY
USING WEIGHT MACHINES

	WEIGHT EXERCISES	DATE:											
1	Bench Press	Weight											
		Reps											
3	Leg Extension	Weight											
		Reps											
5	Lateral Pulldown	Weight											
		Reps											
7	Leg Curl	Weight											
		Reps											
9	Shoulder Press	Weight											
		Reps											
11	Abdominal Curl	Weight											
		Reps											
13	Back Bend	Weight											
		Reps											
15	Leg Press	Weight											
		Reps											
17	Butterfly	Weight											
		Reps											
19	Bicep Curl	Weight											
		Reps											
21	Tricep Curl	Weight											
		Reps											
23	Toe Raises	Reps											
25	Heel Raises	Reps											

NOTE:

- For a Circuit Program, do in sequence 1-25.
- For a Weight Training Program, do odd numbers.
- For an Aerobic Training Program, do even numbers.

	AEROBIC EXERCISES	DATE:										
2	Bike	Time										
4	Ski	Time										
6	Stepper	Time										
8	Treadmill	Time										
10	Jump Rope	Time										
12	Rowing	Time										
14	Bike	Time										
16	Ski	Time										
18	Stepper	Time										
20	Treadmill	Time										
22	Jump Rope	Time										
24	Rowing	Time										

CIRCUIT TRAINING AT HOME

Equipment Requirements:

- 60 minute homemade music tape (60 sec. of music and 15 sec. pause alternating)
- Sturdy straight back chair
- Set of 2-, 5- and 10-lb. hand weights
- Jump rope
- Bench or platform
- Steps or large book

Do each exercise 30-60 seconds and move to the next exercise. You have 15 seconds to accomplish this move. Repeat the circuit until 30 minutes is up. In between each weight or strength exercise, you will jog or ride an exercise bike. You can watch the clock, but one simple way is to make a tape of motivational music. Have a variety of fast paced songs. Play each song for 60 seconds with a 15 second pause. That way you know when to start and finish the exercise.

Circuit Principles

- Select at least one exercise for each major muscle group.
- Spend 30-60 seconds on each exercise.
- Select different aerobic activities (stationary skiing, biking, running in place, etc.)
- Alternate weight lifting with an aerobic activity.
- Allow 15 seconds to change from one activity to another.
- Do 1-3 circuits, depending on your condition.
- Don't lift heavy weights but weights you can do 15-20 times.
- When that weight becomes easy, go to the next level.

Cautions:

- Do at least five minutes of stretching BEFORE and AFTER the circuit.
- When switching from floor to standing exercise, move slowly to prevent dizziness.
- Monitor your heart rate periodically. Strive for at least 65% of your maximum heart rate and no more than 80%.
- If 60 seconds of exercise seems too long, adjust your exercise and rest intervals accordingly (i.e. 30 seconds of exercise and 30 seconds of rest). Gradually work up to 60 seconds of exercise and 15 seconds of rest.

1. **PUSH-UPS:** Keep back straight.

2. **JOG** or use stationary bicycle, ski, rowing machine, or treadmill.

3. **LEG SCISSORS:** Lie on your back with legs in the air and scissor kick side to side. Keep feet off floor.

4. **JOG**

5. **ABDOMINAL CURLS:** Lie on back with knees bent, hands across the chest. Lift shoulders 4"-6" off the floor.

6. **JOG**

7. **ARM CURLS:** Beginners use 2-4 lbs., intermediates 4-8 lbs., advanced use 8-12 lb. weights

8. **JOG**

9. **HALF KNEE BEND:** Do 1/2 squat, rise up on toes with heels raised: then push back up until the legs are straight. Stand flat again. Repeat.

10. **JOG**

11. **TOE RAISES:** Stand with toes on stairs or a large book. Slowly raise up on toes and back down again. Repeat.

12. **JOG**

13. **JUMPING JACKS:** Bring your arms up over your head.

14. **JOG**

15. **CHAIR DIPS:** Sit in chair. Put hands on chair arms and walk forward sliding off seat. Keep legs straight, heels on the floor. Supporting your weight with your arms, lower your body and straighten elbows.

16. **JOG**

17. **SIDE BENDS:** Stand with arms over head. Slowly bend from side to side.

18. **JOG**

19. **SIT UPS:** Hands folded across the chest, knees bent, lift up and touch elbows to respective knees or alternate with left elbow touching right knee one time and right elbow touching left knee the next time.

20. **JOG**

21. **JUMP ROPE**

22. **JOG**

23. **SIDE LEG LIFTS:** Lie on side and lift one leg up away from body. Use ankle weights if desired. Switch sides.

24. **JOG**

25. **STEP UPS:** Step up and down on stairs or bench.

26. **JOG**

27. **CHIN UPS:** Find a strong bar or door to hold on to.

28. **JOG**

END (or start a new circuit)

THE "TRUTH" OF DUMBBELLS

The first two times I heard the "Truth" about dumbbells, I wasn't ready for it. I conducted weight-training workshops at the college. One time Bruce Randall, who became known as the "450 pound fatty who became Mr. Universe" was our speaker. Bruce said he had used dumbbells to reduce his weight to 200 lbs. and win the title in the 1960's. He also was the first weight lifting coach in the NFL with the Washington Redskins.

The second time I heard the "truth" was from another Mr. Universe, Mike Katz, who spoke at a workshop and repeated what Bruce had stated. He said, "If I could only use one piece of equipment to train with, it would be dumbbells."

Dumbbells have many advantages over bar bells and machines. First, they are much easier to store. Second, they don't have the limitations that the bar bells and machines have because there are many more movements and positions you can use. Thirdly, they are much cheaper, and fourth, they are more effective in rehabilitating an injured muscle. For example: for the injured shoulder you can use 5 lbs. and for the good shoulder, 15 or 20 lbs.

Twelve SMART Reasons to Work Out With Dumbbells

1. Dumbbells can give you a more complete workout than any other piece of equipment.

2. You've got a better chance of reaching your long term goals with dumbbells.

3. They're the number one choice for building strength, and they do it faster.

4. They give you a healthier heart.

5. They make your muscles smarter by making them work in three dimensions as opposed to the two dimensions (up & down) of machines.

6. You use them to correct muscle imbalances or rehab injuries.

7. They help prevent injuries. It's easier to injure yourself on a machine.

8. They make the movements safer and more effective because of joint alignment.

9. You can work each muscle from different angles.

10. You can work either unilateral (one side) or bilateral (both sides).

11. They maximize the range of motion, thus improving joint flexibility.

12. You can work out faster with dumbbells than machines, giving you a better aerobic workout.

DON'S DUMBBELL DOZEN

EQUIPMENT REQUIRED:
Set of dumbbells • Flat bench • Exercise mat

NOTE: Take in a DEEP breath when lowering the weight and EXPEL your air on the lift. Before attempting these exercises, first go through using just your body weight. Lift smoothly on a 2 second count, pause and return to start on a 4 second count. Find a weight you can do 7 times and when you can do 12 reps, increase the weight to the next level. Several exercises have different reps listed. Proper form is critical. Do each exercise in a slow, controlled manner.

> **VERSATILE DUMBBELLS:**
> SPRI Products has a 30 lb. adjustable chrome dumbell set in a carrying case for $50. (1-800-222-7774)

1. **LUNGE** — Quads and Hams (15 reps)
   • Stand with back straight, head up, feet 6" apart, dumbbells by side, palms in.
   • Holding weight at your side, keeping right leg straight, take step forward with left leg. (You should end up with left thigh almost parallel to the floor)
   • Reverse the motion, stepping back to the starting position.
   • Inhale as you lunge, exhale as you return.
   • Repeat with the right leg.

2. **CHEST PRESS** — Pecs and Delts
   • With dumbbell in each hand, lie on the bench, feet flat on the floor.
   • Start with weights at chest level, next to the shoulders, palms facing forward.
   • Push the dumbbells toward the ceiling.
   • At the top of the extension, keep elbows slightly bent.
   • Return to chest in slow motion.

3. **ONE LEG CALF RAISE** — (15 reps each leg)
   • Hold dumbbell at left side with palm against the leg.
   • Step on secure platform, heels hanging off the edge. Put weight on balls of feet.
   • Place your right hand against wall or railing for support.
   • Tuck your right foot behind your left heel.
   • With your head and back straight, rise up on the toes of your left foot.
   • After 15 reps, switch the weight to the right side and use your right leg.

4. **SEATED MILITARY PRESS** — Delts
   - Have your back slightly arched and feet on the floor.
   - Raise the weights from your shoulder up with the palms facing forward.
   - Don't lock the elbows and lower weights under control.

5A. **ABDOMINAL CRUNCH** — Basic (Build up to 25)
   - Lie on rug on the floor with knees bent, arms folded across your chest and lower back pressed against the floor.
   - Slowly roll upper body forward until shoulder blades are 4-6" off floor.
   - Pause and slowly roll back to starting position.

5B. **ABDOMINAL CRUNCH, ADVANCED** — (Build up to 25 reps)
   - Lie on your back with knees bent and calves draped over an exercise bench.
   - Fold your arms across your chest.
   - Keep your head tucked slightly in toward the chest and slowly curl your upper body toward your legs until your shoulder blades come 4-6" off the floor.
   - Hold for a couple of seconds before slowly returning to starting position. If this becomes easy, cradle a 5 to 25 pound weight plate across your chest.

6. **STANDING UPRIGHT ROW** — Shoulders/Neck/Back
   - Hold pair of Dumbbells against the front of thighs
   - Lift the weights, keeping them close to the body until they're just below your chin.
   - Hold for 2 seconds and slowly lower to starting position.

7. **OVERHEAD ELBOW EXTENSION** — Triceps
   - Hold dumbbell in one hand, held behind the back of the neck, directly in line with the shoulders.
   - With opposite hand, grasp under the elbow for stability.
   - Extend the elbow until the arm is fully extended above the head.
   - Pause and return to starting position.

8. **SIDE BEND** — Obliques
   - Hold dumbbell in left hand at side.
   - Place right hand on waist.
   - Slowly bend to left as far as you can.
   - Slowly return to standing and bend right.
   - Do 15 reps.
   - Switch dumbbell to right hand and repeat.

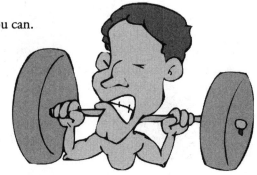

9. **DEADLIFT** — Glutes, Quads, Lower Back
   - Stand with feet shoulder width, dumbbells in front of thighs, palms in.
   - Bend over at waist to 90 degrees. Keeping back flat, not rounded, lower weights down leg.
   - Raise back up slowly to full extension, keeping elbows locked in, weights close to leg.

10. **BENT ARM LATERAL RAISE** — Shoulders
    - Stand with feet shoulder width apart.
    - Hold dumbbells at sides, palms facing in.
    - Raise arms straight out to sides to shoulder level, palms facing floor.
    - Lower arms to starting position.

11. **STANDING CURLS** — Biceps
    - Stand erect, a dumbbell in each hand, palms facing forward, arms down at your sides.
    - Bend elbows and curl the weights to shoulder height.
    - Hold 2 seconds and reverse the motion.

12. **WRIST CURL** — (15 reps)
    - Sit on bench with knees shoulder width and feet flat on floor.
    - With dumbbells in each hand (palms up), lean forward, placing forearm across thigh.
    - Allow knuckles to drop in front of knees.
    - Slowly lift the weight with only hands and wrists.
    - Do one set with palms up and second set with palms facing downward.

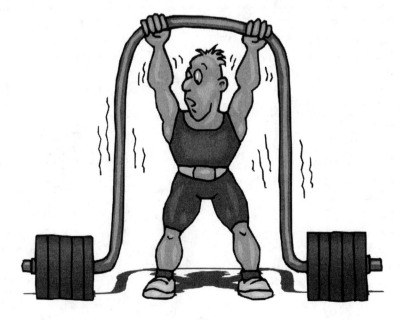

85

DUMBBELL DOZEN

TIP: *To protect your back, use proper lifting technique to pick up dumbbells from the floor. Bend at the knees (not at the waist) and rise slowly.*

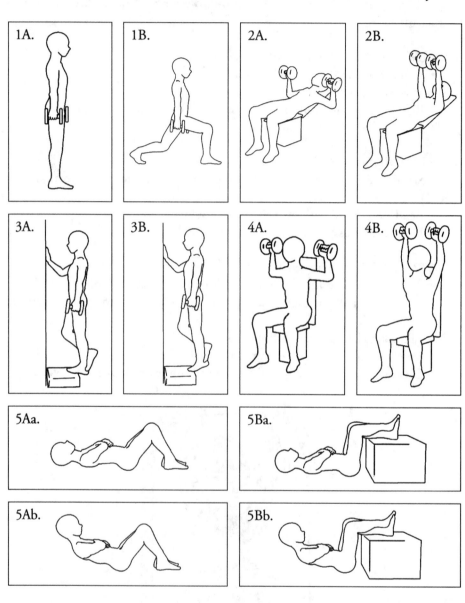

1A / 1B	Lunge	4A / 4B	Seated Military Press
2A / 2B	Chest Press	5Aa / 5Ab	Crunch – Basic
3A / 3B	One Leg Calf Raise	5Ba / 5Bb	Crunch – Advanced

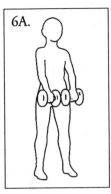

6A.

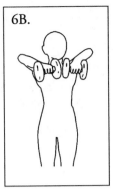

6B.

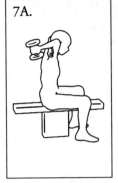

7A.

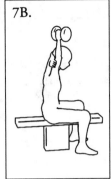

7B.

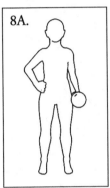

8A.

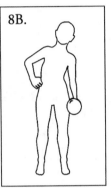

8B.

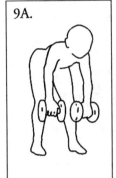

9A.

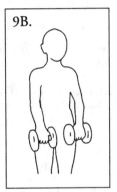

9B.

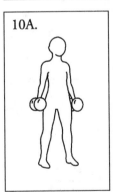

10A.

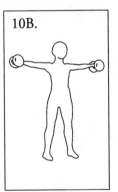

10B.

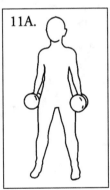

11A.

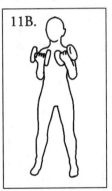

11B.

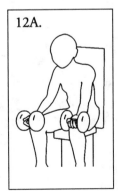

12A.

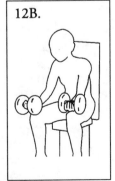

12B.

6A / 6B	Standing Upright Row
7A / 7B	Seated Triceps Curl
8A / 8B	Side Bend
9A / 9B	Dead Lift
10A / 10B	Bent Arm Lateral Raise
11A / 11B	Standing Curls
12A / 12B	Wrist Curl

PERSONAL TRAINER WORKOUT

Most of us can't afford the services of a personal trainer on a regular basis, but periodically it is a good practice. Here are samples of two personal trainer workouts. Of course, the trainer would personalize the workout according to your fitness level.

60 Minute Workout

- 5-10 min. warm-up (stationary bike, walking, stair machine, stretching).
- 30 min. weight resistance (one set, 10-12 rep each of 10-15 exercises).
- 20 minutes cardiovascular training (treadmill, bike, rower, stepper).
- Cool down and full body stretch.

90 Minute Workout

- 5 min. warm-up (same as above).
- 5-10 min. full body stretches.
- 15 min. abdominal workout.
- 45 min. chest/triceps and leg workout.
- 15-20 min. cardiovascular training (treadmill, bike, rower)
- Cool down and full body stretch.

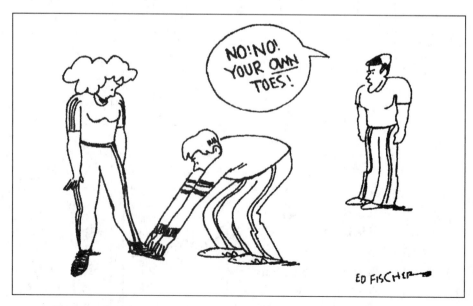

(Reprinted with permission from Dr. Jeff Haebig, Wellness Quest©)

BANDS AND TUBING

Bands and tubing have been used for years in the physical therapy fields to rehabilitate, strengthen, and condition injured muscles. After several studies showed that bands can be used to strengthen healthy muscles, they have become very popular, particularly for those who do a lot of traveling. They take up less room in your suitcase than a pair of socks and their cost is only $10 to $15. Studies have shown that they compare favorably with weight machines and free weights.

One system I like is the "Stretch For Strength" system designed by Rob Sweetgall. This features tubing with handles with three strength levels: weak, medium and strong. It comes complete with illustrated manual. When the 10th repetition becomes easy, then it is time to move up to a stronger resistance. Conversely, if it is difficult to do 4-5 reps., then you need to switch to a lower resistance. You can do squats, biceps curls, chest press, leg presses, leg curls, leg extension, lateral pull-downs, seated rows, hamstring curls, and much more, and you can do them in the comfort of your living room or hotel room.

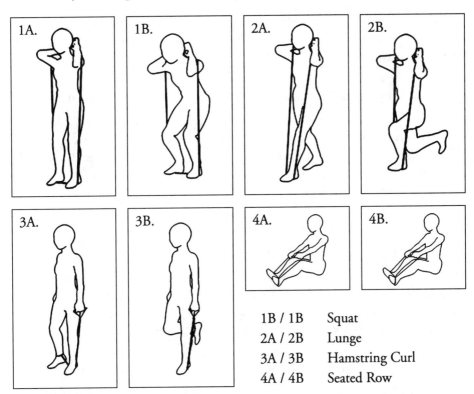

1B / 1B	Squat
2A / 2B	Lunge
3A / 3B	Hamstring Curl
4A / 4B	Seated Row

To purchase the "Stretch for Strength" System call Rainbow Wellness: 269-925-3524.

SOME STRENGTH TRAINING MYTHS

MYTH: If you lift weights you will bulk up and become "muscle bound."

FACT: It's physiologically impossible for women to build "Schwarzenegger" sized biceps. For that matter, very few men can do it. They just don't have the necessary genetics. Besides, since muscle is denser than fat and has definition, strength training makes muscles shapelier.

MYTH: You can spot reduce and lose saddlebags and unwanted bulges.

FACT: There is no such thing as "spot" reduction. Area specific exercises can improve appearance by tightening underlying muscle, but it's fantasy to think you can choose where to burn fat. The general rule is that fat comes off in the reverse order that it was put on. Last on, first off.

MYTH: In order to see results, you need to work every muscle individually.

FACT: You get a more efficient workout by performing compound moves, i.e. squats, lunges, dips and pushups.

MYTH: To increase muscle size, you need extra protein.

FACT: The RDA requirement for protein is .8 g. for each 2.2 lbs. (1 kg) of weight. For a 150 lb. person, this translates into about 55 grams of protein. For a 200 lb. person, it is 72 grams. For athletes, the number is only slightly higher at 1 gram per 2.2 lbs or 90 grams for the 200 lb. athlete. The liver and kidneys can only assimilate so much protein. The excess is excreted as urine.

MYTH: For maximum muscle definition (tone), you need to do a lot of repetitions.

FACT: The only way you'll see gains in muscle size or strength, is to take the muscle to momentary muscle failure (usually 10-15 reps.) by using the principle of progressive resistance as explained earlier in this chapter. If repetitions produced large biceps, carpenters who pound nails all day long would have 22 inch biceps.

MYTH: If you stop working out, your muscles will turn to fat.

FACT: That's like saying that you can turn an orange into an apple. Muscle and fat are two different substances. Stop working out and your body becomes less efficient at burning calories, thus pounds of fat appear and your muscles atrophy through disuse. "Use it or lose it."

CHAPTER SIX:
WALKING, AQUASIZING AND SWIMMING

THIS IS EXERCISE?

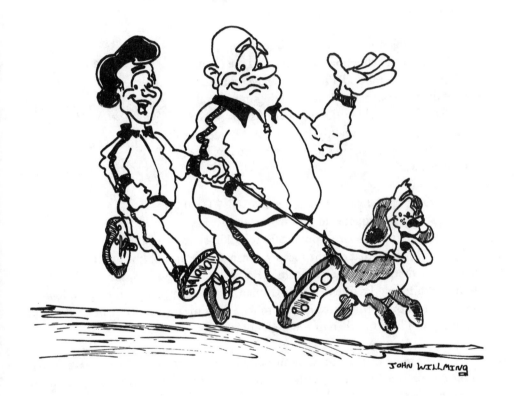

"Walk as though you have a place to go."

"Take a two mile walk every morning before breakfast."

— Harry S. Truman

WALKING, AQUASIZING AND SWIMMING

10,000 Steps ... A Magic Number?

For most people, walking is an ideal aerobic activity. If you are not disabled, you can walk, whatever your age or muscle state. Walking for exercise is as near as the front door; it requires no special equipment, no lessons with a pro, and no large expenditure beyond the price of a good pair of walking shoes. Walking is the cheapest exercise in time, money, and energy. It is the most accessible and most generally available form of exercise. Most fitness experts list walking as one of the best forms of exercise.

The Cooper Institute for Aerobic Research of Dallas, TX, the Stanford School of Medicine, and the Centers for Disease Control and Prevention have conducted studies on fitness in general, and walking in particular. They have been tracking the number of steps per day required to meet the Healthy People 2000 guidelines of accumulating 30 minutes of moderate activity, most days of the week.

> *....walking is an ideal aerobic activity. The goal is to walk 10,000 steps a day.*

Their research indicates that people need to walk 10,000 steps a day, which equates to approximately 5 miles. A mile of walking can vary from 1,800 to 2,200 steps depending on stride length and pace. However, that doesn't mean you can shuffle around the house doing light domestic activities or light gardening. Rather, it is to walk briskly. One rule of thumb is to follow President Harry Truman's walking style, which he described as "walking as though I have someplace to go." This means that your heart rate and breathing will be faster than during lighter activities.

Most people move through life walking without a fitness purpose. The average person in the course of a normal day walks 3,000 to 5,000. I have purchased a pedometer that is highly sophisticated. It keeps track of the number of steps, distance covered, and calories burned (based on my body weight). It is called the Digi Walker.

I have been fascinated by how motivational this small, lightweight device is. On the days that I get no "formal" exercise, I'm lucky to accumulate 3,000 steps. On the days I go for a 3 mile walk on my home treadmill or outside (which I prefer when the weather is good), I come close to 10,000. On the days that I play badminton or tennis and walk, I've accumulated as much as 17,000 steps. One day I had 5,000 steps in a 2 hour tennis doubles match.

TOTAL BODY WORKOUT

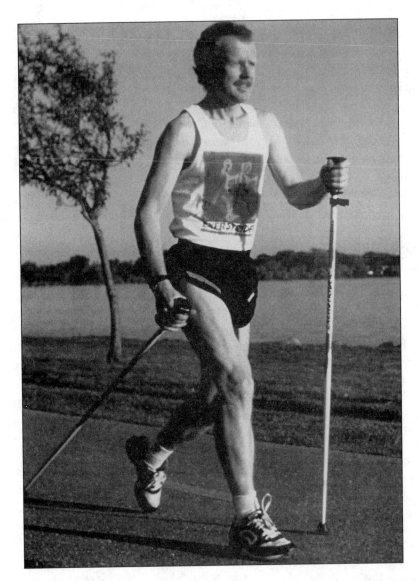

Tom Rutlin, founder/inventor of Exerstrider Walking Poles demonstrating correct technique.

EXERSTRIDING: Exerstriding transforms walking into a total body exercise. By using light weight poles (similar to ski poles), the arms, stomach, chest, and back muscles contribute to a 30-50% increase in exercise intensity compared to regular walking. An added benefit is that the poles reduce stress on the leg joints. This makes them desirable for people with arthritis and other joint problems.

FOR INFORMATION ON OBTAINING EXERSTRIDERS CALL 269-925-3524.

GET A PROGRAM, NOT JUST A PEDOMETER

Rob Sweetgall, America's leading advocate of walking for wellness, has put together a Digi Walker kit. It includes a manual called "Pedometer Walking" with a variety of walking programs, a walking text and 52 weeks of walking logs. The entire kit of the Digi Walker, manual and tape for measuring the length of your steps costs $30. Individual books are available for $10. For information on the Digi Walker Kit, call Rainbow Wellness: 269-925-3524.

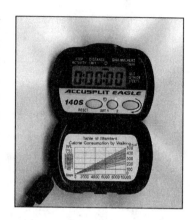

Basic Walking Categories

STROLLING: (20-30 MINUTE MILE). Research shows health is improved anytime you move or do more physical work than you are used to-if you do it consistently. So, if you have never exercised, strolling, especially with friends, is the place to start! Strolling does not maximize cardiovascular fitness, BUT we hope you'll feel so much better you'll progress to fitness walking. Examples of strolling are shopping, walking with kids, neighborhood or lunch time strolls with friends.

FITNESS WALKING: (12-20 MINUTE MILE). With fitness walking, you will achieve health benefits if you walk often enough (Frequency), fast enough (Intensity), long enough (Time), and do it with a friend (Social) FITS.

POWER WALKING: (10-12 MINUTE MILE). Power walking is similar to fitness walking but the length and frequency of your stride(s) is increased. The speed and intensity this adds to your workout enhances your fitness levels.

CALORIC EXPENDITURE		
PACE	WALKING	EXERSTRIDERS
3.0 mph	4.0 cal. per minute	5.5 cal. per minute
3.5 mph	5.0 cal. per minute	7.0 cal. per minute
4.0 mph	6.0 cal. per minute	8.5 cal. per minute

Based on 150 lb. person

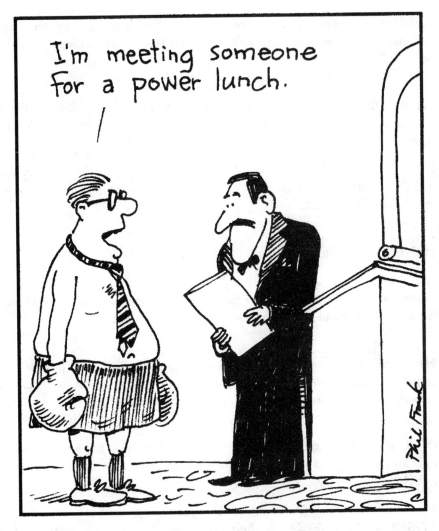

Walking is such an easy activity that you don't need a long warm up. However, a short warm up will help you perform better and decrease the slight aches and pains most people experience with a new exercise program.

A warm-up is particularly important if you exercise first thing in the morning or after sitting in your office all day. You can begin your warm up by walking at a slower pace for the first quarter of a mile then stopping for a few minutes to do stretches.

CAUTION: DO NOT BOUNCE WHEN DOING STRETCHES.
For stretches, see chapter 4

TECHNIQUES FOR FITNESS WALKING

- **POSTURE** — Good posture is important. Walk with the chin up, shoulders, back and chest lifted, and hips under shoulders (body does not lean forward or backward). "Think tall."

- **SHOULDERS** — Shoulders should be square to the direction of travel and be relaxed. Keep them close to the body. Swing arms front to back, not across the body.

- **ARMS** — Arms should be bent 90° at the elbow swinging in a relaxed yet vigorous manner.

- **HANDS** — Hold in line with wrist and a lightly closed fist.

- **HIP MOVEMENT** — Hips rotate forward at waist with the lead leg lengthening the stride. Hips should not wiggle or twist from side to side.

- **FOOT ACTION** — As the foot strikes the ground, the heel is placed down and the foot rolls forward to the toe along the outside edge of the foot. Push-off powerfully by aggressively extending the back leg and foot.

- **OPPOSITION** — Swing your arms in opposition to your leg movements, i.e. right arm goes forward as left leg goes forward and visa versa with the left arm and right leg.

- **STRIDE** — Walk briskly, but don't over stride. To increase your speed, take shorter and quicker steps.

"Tis the best of humanity that comes out to walk."

— Ralph Waldo Emerson

WALKING ANALYSIS

Name _____ Evaluator _____

Correct walking posture helps boost calorie burn and prevent injuries. To check your technique, have a friend watch you walk. These are the keys to good walking posture.

	YES	NO
LEVEL HEAD:		
Look 8-10 feet forward	___	___
Chin is parallel to ground	___	___
Ears should be over the shoulders	___	___
LEVEL SHOULDERS:		
No slouching	___	___
Relaxed neck and back	___	___
Square to the direction of travel	___	___
ARM SWING:		
Arms bent 80-90 degrees at elbow	___	___
Do not pump arms – swing in relaxed manner	___	___
No higher than breast bone	___	___
Close to the side of the body	___	___
Elbows near waist	___	___
Hands stay below chest level	___	___
Swing arms in opposition to legs (left arm, right leg)	___	___
HIP MOVEMENT:		
Hips should not wiggle from side to side	___	___
POSTURE:		
Walk tall	___	___
Point knees and toes forward	___	___
FEET:		
Straight ahead – no pigeon toed or duck feet	___	___
Walking on a narrow line	___	___
Push off with back foot	___	___
HEEL/TOE: (HEEL, BALL AND TOE)		
Land on heel	___	___
Transfer weight to ball	___	___
Push off your toes	___	___
FORWARD LEAN:		
Slight lean forward from ankles, no waist	___	___
Don't reach or lunge with your foot	___	___
STRIDE:		
No bouncing stride	___	___
Push forward, not up	___	___
Walk briskly, quick steps	___	___

SUGGESTIONS BEFORE STARTING
A WALKING PROGRAM

1. **HAVE A GOAL:** A good goal to start with is to walk at least 30 minutes a day, five days a week. As you get in better shape, aim for a longer time.

2. **MAKE A DAILY APPOINTMENT WITH YOURSELF:** Set a time and don't let anything interfere with it.

3. **BE REALISTIC IN YOUR EXPECTATIONS:** If you know that you have low aerobic conditioning, start out with the strolling program.

4. **DETERMINE YOUR LEVEL:** Use the walking test that follows to determine your starting level.

5. **WALK WITH A BUDDY:** Support works!

6. **CHOOSE SHOES WISELY:** Use good shoes that have the proper support to prevent muscle and joint injuries. Although you won't experience the joint stresses you might get if you were running, you still exert a significant force each time your foot hits the pavement. If you are not familiar with shoes designed for walking for exercise, ask for assistance at a store that specializes in running/walking gear. They will want to see the shoes you currently walk in to determine the strike pattern of your stride. Most will advise an economical but efficient shoe that has a firm heel cup for stability, a rocker sole to enhance a smooth heel-to-toe motion, and plenty of room for the toes to spread out as you push off. Be sure to try on both shoes using the athletic socks you will use during walking. Walk around the store to assess comfort. Many people prefer running shoes for walking.

7. **MONITOR YOUR PROGRESS:** Use a journal or log book to keep track of your walking.

8. **TAKE A CHALLENGE:** Consider enrolling in the President's Sports and Fitness Awards program. (www.presidentschallenge.org)

Determining Your Starting Level

Before you begin any exercise program, review the medical history questionnaire provided at the beginning of this book. Then take the Walking Test described on the next page to assure that you start at a realistic level.

FITNESS WALKING TEST

To Take This Test You Will Need:

- to be able to monitor your heart rate (pulse). (see instructions below)

- the chart on the worksheet with this program.

- a track or any flat surfaced road that has a measured mile.

- clothing that is comfortable (layering clothes is smart because the test will make you warm).

> *"To improve aerobic fitness, you need to walk at least 30 minutes a day, 5 days a week."*
>
> — *US Surgeon General*

Before You Start: *Practice monitoring your pulse:*

- Walk in place for 30 seconds.

- Lightly place your second and third fingers on the inside of your wrist until you feel your pulse.

- Count your pulse for 15 seconds.

- To get your heart rate per minute, multiply this number by 4.

- An alternative location to monitor your pulse is on the side of your neck next to your Adam's apple and below your jaw.

- Practice using a stopwatch or have a buddy who can keep time for you.

Taking The Test:

- Note the starting time.

- Briskly walk one mile, trying to maintain an even pace.

- As soon as you finish the mile, make a note of how long it took.

- Immediately take your pulse for 15 seconds (since it will drop rapidly when you quit walking).

- Multiply the result of your pulse check by 4 to get a one minute pulse.

- Record your walking time and your one minute pulse.

- Determine your fitness category from the following graph.

HOW TO DETERMINE YOUR FITNESS LEVEL:

1. Find your age category in the charts below.
2. On the bottom line, locate the time it took you to walk one mile.
3. On the left line, locate your heart rate.
4. From each of these points, draw a line across the chart. The point where these two lines intersect is your fitness level.

For example: If you are 45 years old, have a 14 minute time and a heart rate of 150, you're in the "good" category.

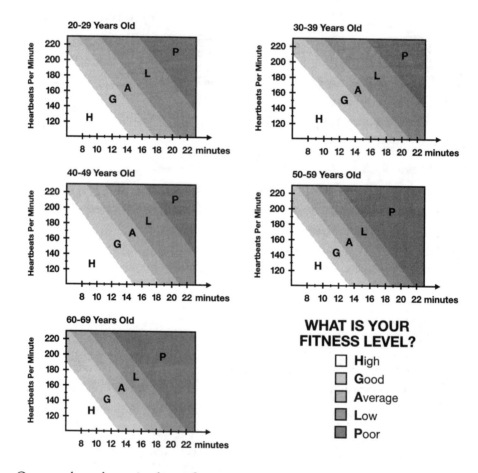

Once you have determined your fitness category, you will know which level to begin. For example, if you were in the average fitness category, you would start out with 40 minutes of walking at 3 mph or 20 minute miles At this rate, you would cover 2 miles daily, or 10 miles weekly. At the end of the fourth and eighth weeks, repeat the "Fitness Walking Test" and move to the appropriate fitness level.

WALKING PROGRAM: Personal Fitness Level

	1ST TEST	2ND TEST	3RD TEST
Date			
Pulse (60 sec.)	bpm	bpm	bpm
Walking Time	min.	min.	min.
Fitness Category			

WALKING PROGRAM: Based on Your Fitness Level

FITNESS CATEGORY	WALKING TIME	SPEED	DAILY DISTANCE	WEEKLY DISTANCE
Poor	30 min. at	3.0 mph	1.5 mi.	7.5 mi.
Low	35 min. at	3.0 mph	1.75 mi.	8.75 mi.
Average	40 min. at	3.0 mph	2.0 mi.	10 mi.
Good	45 min. at	3.5 mph	2.6 mi.	13 mi.
High	50 min. at	4.0-4.5 mph	3.0-4.0 mi.	15-2 mi.

If you feel like doing more than the above, increase time and distance, but don't increase the walking speed without doing another test to determine your fitness level. As a general rule, the walking speed should increase about 1/2 mile per hour every 4 weeks. That means that you can go from the low or average category to high category in 8-10 weeks.

MOTIVATIONAL TIP:

If a person were to adopt walking as a lifetime activity and walk daily for 60 minutes at a fitness pace, in one year they could lose over 30 lbs.

STEP UP TO VOLKSWALKING

Volkswalks originated in Germany and were imported to the United States in 1979. They are designed to be community or family walks.

Volkswalks, or "people's walks," are:

- Non-competitive events – not tests of speed or endurance. Participants walk at their own pace and can stop to rest, sightsee, or picnic.

- There are walking, swimming, biking, and cross country skiing events.

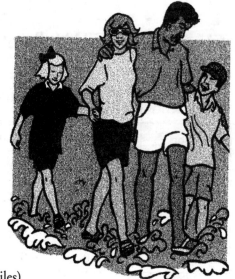

- It is based on the belief that everyone should be encouraged to exercise and receive a medal or ribbon, regardless of their placing or time.

- There are over 550 AVA clubs and 1,200 walks held annually in the United States.

- Volkswalks are normally 10 km (6.2 miles) walks and usually cover historical sites like Gettysburg; Mount Vernon; Mackinac Island; Ft. Sam Houston; Concord, MA; Virginia City, NV; Greenfield Village, MI; West Point; Washington DC Monument Walk, and many more.

- Others are scenic such as Carmel, CA; Diamond Head, Hawaii; Garden of the Gods, CO; San Antonio Riverwalk; Central Park, NY; Notre Dame University; or along Lake Michigan in St. Joseph, MI.

- Most Volkswalks are year around events.

If you are interested in more information about Volkswalks, contact the AVA at 210-659-2112 or www.ava.org.

TREADMILL: GOING NOWHERE FAST

"There's more to treadmill walking
than putting one foot in front of the other."

The treadmill has become the most effective piece of fitness equipment for strengthening the heart, increasing endurance, burning fat, toning muscles, reducing stress, and improving mood — all in the boundaries of your home.

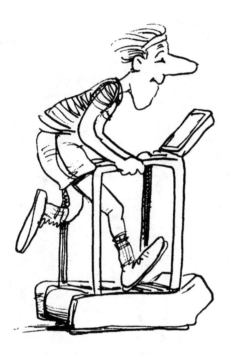

A study reported in the American Medical Journal determined that of the following six exercise machines: stepper, treadmill, bicycle, rower, air dyne, and ski machine, the treadmill workout was the most effective in terms of caloric expenditure.

In spite of jokes about going nowhere fast, there are many ways to energize your workout, such as listening to music or an educational tape, watching TV, or reading. Most of us, if given the choice, would prefer to walk outdoors, but many times it's too hot, too cold, too icy, too dangerous, too late at night, etc.

The advantage of the treadmill is that you can increase the intensity of the workout two ways: by raising the elevation and/or increasing the speed. For every degree of increase in elevation (with no increase in speed), you'll increase the heart rate by 3-5 beats per minute and increase the caloric expenditure. By walking at a 5 degree elevation, you can raise your heart rate 15-25 bpm and increase the caloric expenditure by 30-40%. You can also increase the intensity by increasing your speed. Going from 3 mph (142 calories) to 4 mph (279 calories) you can increase the "burn" by over 50%.

Treadmills "Burn" Calories Best

Treadmill	700 cph*
Stairmaster	627 cph
Rower	606 cph
Skiing Machine	595 cph
Air Dyne	509 cph
Stationary Bike	498 cph

* cph = calories per hour
Study by Medical College of WI

TREADMILL CALORIC EXPENDITURE IS A FUNCTION OF ELEVATION AND SPEED.

The following figures are based on a 30 minute workout for a 175 lb. person

ELEVATION	SPEED	CALORIES EXPENDED
0°	3 MPH	142
5°	4 MPH	279
10°	5 MPH	547

You can see that you can go from an expenditure of 142 calories to 547 calories for a 30 minute workout just by increasing the speed and elevation. This same analogy applies to walking outside on flat ground or hills. CAUTION: Should you feel any discomfort during any treadmill workout, stop immediately. These are warning signs that need to be discussed with your doctor.

Treadmill Do's and Don'ts

DO   Walk with each foot pointed ahead.

DO   Keep your trunk motionless, not swaying your torso or bobbing your head.

DON'T   Walk hunched over the rail; use the handrail only if necessary for balance.

DON'T   Carry hand weights or wear leg weights.

BUYING POWER

Here are four features to look for when buying a treadmill:

1. Lots of room to walk. A walking surface shorter than 50 inches and 18 inches wide will be too small.

2. Plenty of speed. A maximum of 8-10 mph is a must.

3. Inclines are a must. You should have at least a 10% incline capability.

4. The more power the better. Look for a motor rated at least 2.0 horsepower continuous duty. Anything less and you will have rougher rides, more frequent trips to the repair shop and a shorter treadmill life.

Why They Run

For every runner who tours the world running marathons,

there are thousands who run to hear the leaves and listen

to the rain, and look to the day when it is suddenly as easy

as a bird in flight. For them, sport is not a test but a therapy,

not a trial but a reward, not a question but an answer.

— George Sheehan, M.D. noted runner, author and teacher

*Author's note: you can substitute walker, swimmer, etc. for the word, runner

REMEMBERING GEORGE SHEEHAN

In the 1970's and 1980's, my favorite writer and speaker was the cardiologist, marathon runner George Sheehan. I had the privilege of listening to Dr. Sheehan speak on many occasions, and I would always read his monthly column in "Runners World." He was a prolific writer, and I have several of his books (autographed). George always made you think; therefore, he was called the "Walter Thoreau of running."

In 1986 he learned that he had prostate cancer. At first he surrendered to the disease. He stopped running, writing, and accepting speaking engagements. But this didn't last long. He soon realized that waiting to die was no way to spend his remaining time. He wrote, "There is nothing more certain than the defeat of a man who gives up-and, I might add, the victory of one who will not."

He resumed his full menu of writing, running (which later turned into walking), delivering hundreds of speeches, running races, writing columns and publishing two more books. More importantly, he patched up his personal life by ending a long separation from his wife and their 12 children.

In 1992 he was forced to put an end to his running and speaking but he continued to write until his death November 1, 1993. On the 10 year anniversary of George's death, Joe Henderson, long time editor and personal friend of his, released the unpublished essay on running that George had written in June 1993.

NOTE: This is the last article Dr. Sheehan wrote before his death in November 1993. It wasn't published until December 2003

WHY DO I RUN?

By George Sheehan

I have written over the years of the benefits I receive from running. Enumerated the physical and mental changes. Listed the emotional and spiritual gains. Charted the improvement that has taken place in my person and my life. What I have not emphasized is how transient these values and virtues are.

With just a little thought, however, it should be evident that physical laws parallel those of the mind and the spirit. We know that the effects of training are temporary. I cannot put fitness in the bank. If inactive, I will detrain faster than it took me to get in shape. And since my entire persona is influenced by my running program, I must remain constantly in training. Otherwise, the sedentary life will inexorably reduce my mental and emotional well-being.

So I run each day to preserve the self I attained the day before. And coupled with this is the desire to secure the self yet to be. There can be no let up. If I do not run, I will eventually lose all I have gained-and my future with it.

Maintenance was a favorite topic of writer and philosopher Erik Hoffer. It made the difference, said the former longshoreman, between a country that was successful and one that failed. An achievement, no matter how magnificent, will eventually decay if not preserved by constant care. I know that experience intimately. There is nothing briefer than the winner's laurel. Victory is of the moment. It must be followed by another victory and then another. I have to run just to stay in place.

Excellence is not something attained and put in a trophy case. It is not sought after, achieved, and thereafter, a steady state. It is a momentary phenomenon, a rare conjunction of body, mind, and spirit at one's peak. Should I come to that peak, I cannot stay there. Like Sisyphus, I must start each day at the bottom and work back up to the top. And then beyond that peak to another and yet another.

Through running I have learned what I can be and do. My body is now sensitive to the slightest change. It is particularly aware of any decline or decay. I can feel this lessening of the "me" that I have come to think of myself.

Running has made this new me. Taken the raw material and honed it and delivered it back ready to do the work of a human being. I run so I do not lose the me I was yesterday and the me I might become tomorrow. (Henderson 61)

WATER WORKOUTS

The Pool Offers an Alternative to the Gym

Water fitness programs have evolved beyond monotonous laps with kick boards or rubber tubes around your legs to a fun way to stay in shape. Swimming has become a popular cross training activity. Triathlons (swimming, biking, and running) are also more popular now.

The same thing is true of water aerobics or aquacising. These used to have the reputation of being an "old people's workout." Not anymore! Water aerobics combines all five aspects of fitness: cardiovascular, muscular strength and endurance, flexibility, and weight control. The beauty of water aerobics is that you don't have to know anything about swimming as you can do an entire workout in water that is chest high. You can even do a workout without getting your hair wet!

The best aspect of a water workout is that you can tailor the intensity of the workout to match your fitness level. If you have movement limitations from arthritis or injury, the warm water will serve as therapy, while you rehabilitate your muscles. Both times before my hip replacements, I was in the water right up until the surgery and within two weeks afterwards. NOTE: If you are using the water for therapy, look for the water temperature to be 84 degrees or above.

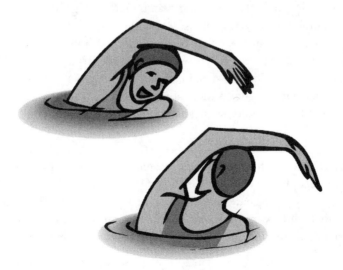

If you're a serious exerciser, looking for an intense workout, you can get that also. With a swim belt, empty milk containers or a noodle (a long foam cylinder that can be bent or twisted) you can race walk, run, cross country ski, bicycle, and do crunches in the deep water. Practically anything you do on land you can duplicate in the water. Since the water provides 12-14% more resistance than air, you can get as strenuous a workout as you desire, without it becoming a weight bearing exercise.

You can do water aerobics or swim. Both choices will give you a great workout.

EXERCISE HEART RATE FOR SWIMMING

A general rule is that the swimming heart rate is typically 10 to 20 beats per minute less than what it is for dry land activity. Use the "Perceived exertion test." If it feels somewhat hard to hard, then you're in the Target Heart Rate.

SWIMMING

Swimming is considered, by most fitness experts, as one of the top four cardiovascular activities. These four, in order of benefits are: running, cross-country skiing, swimming, and fitness walking. The ideal fitness program would be to incorporate at least three of these activities in your workout routine, particularly swimming. As we get older (everyone is getting older!), swimming stands out as a good choice for a number of reasons. First, there is no weight on your joints when you're in the water. Second, by combining arms and legs you get a great total body workout. Third, varying your strokes, i.e. breast, side, crawl and back-strokes is a good way to improve your flexibility. Using a variety of equipment such as kick boards, fins, and hand-paddles, you can vary the intensity of your workout.

One caveat: If your main goal is to lose weight, don't expect swimming to be the answer. Many people in "Dump Your Plump™" use swimming as their mode of exercise, and they've had a hard time making their weight goals. Fitness experts have determined that while swimming is one of the best cardiovascular exercises, it burns fewer calories than running and other weight bearing activities.

There are several interesting theories about why this is so. According to Jane Van Heest, Ph.D., director of exercise physiology for United States Swimming, the reason may be that extra body fat is not an advantage for a runner, but for a swimmer, body fat acts as a flotation aid increasing buoyancy. Also, fat helps keep the body insulated from cool water. However, she points out that this theory is based on observation and has never been proven.

In the 1980's, I recall asking Covert Bailey, at one of his "Fit or Fat" workshops, why swimmers carried extra weight and his answer was, "You've never seen a skinny whale, have you?" Maybe there is some truth in his flippant reply.

If you are not a very proficient swimmer, consider investing in some lessons. You will be glad many times over for doing this, as you lose motivation quickly if you have poor stroking technique. Lessons are readily available at the YMCA's, schools, and fitness clubs.

FINDING A POOL WHEN TRAVELING

This can be difficult. Usually when the hotel has a pool, it's too small for laps or too crowded with kids. Go to www.swimmersguide.com before you hit the road to find pools conducive to lap swimming.

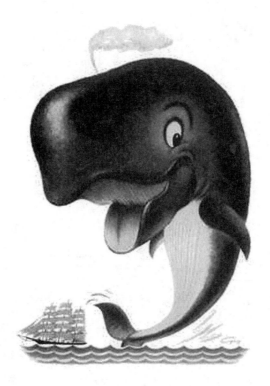

AQUA AEROBICS

Listed below are samples of different water exercises.

WARM UP/ COOL DOWN

Side Stretch
Lunge Stretch
Knee Raise and Hold
Body Turns
Trunk Twists
Skiers Stretch
Stretch Up
Shoulder stretch
Head Turns
Walking
Arm Circles

WALL EXERCISES

Wall Lunges
Walk the Wall
Leg Lifts
Leg Circles
Burpees
Front Push ups
Back Push ups
Hinge Kicks
Wall Sit Ups
Back/Front Flutter
Pendulum Leg Swing
Bicycle
Knee Tucks
Scissor Kick
V legs
Leg Swing

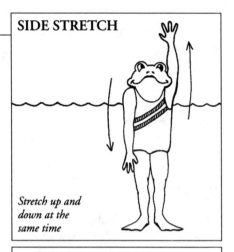

SIDE STRETCH

Stretch up and down at the same time

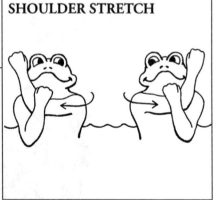

SHOULDER STRETCH

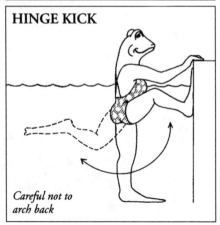

HINGE KICK

Careful not to arch back

AEROBIC

Jumping Jack
Cross country Ski
Twist & Jump
Russian Dance
Rope Skipping
Punch Up, Out, Down
Jog in Place
Boxers Crossover
Side to Side Lunges
Walk/Run Across Pool
March in Place
Side to Side Lunges
Bicycle – deep water
Sit-ups – deep water
Jog – deep water

*Illustrations: Courtesy of
Judy Davenport Conley,
Water Aerobics Instructor
www.waterart.org.*

"V" LEGS

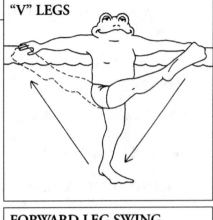

FORWARD LEG SWING

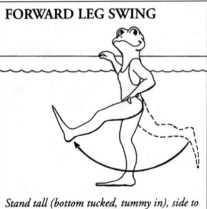

*Stand tall (bottom tucked, tummy in), side to
wall. Swing outside leg forward and back.*

UP-SIDE-DOWN

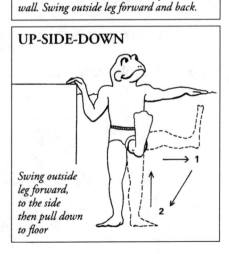

*Swing outside
leg forward,
to the side
then pull down
to floor*

BASIC TIPS FOR SWIMMING THE CRAWL

1. **CONCENTRATE ON UPPER BODY,** not lower. The crawl is 75% upper body work.

2. **LENGTHEN YOUR BODY.** Extend your arm with an open hand and grab "fresh" water, not water already in motion. Extend the arm until the shoulder touches the jaw.

3. **RAISE YOUR ELBOWS.** Keep your elbows higher than your hand so your fingers enter the water first.

4. **FORM AN S.** As you pull your right arm through the water, form an inverted S shape. Form a normal S as you maneuver the left are. Don't drag your arms through the water in a straight line. Finish with the hand brushing the thigh.

5. **ROLL YOUR HEAD.** Don't lift the head out of the water to breathe, roll it to the side.

6. **KICK.**
   a. Keep your knees straight during the upward kick.
   b. Keep the knees slightly bent during the downward kick.
   c. Keep the ankles flexible - never from the knees.
   d. Kick from the hip - never from the knees.
   e. Don't kick higher than the water surface or lower than the lowest part of your body.
   f. Use the two beat kick - one leg stroke to one arm stroke.

7. **HIDE YOUR HEAD.** Lead with the top of your head - not your forehead. Look at the bottom of the pool.

8. **FLOW LIKE WATER.** Be quiet with your body. Waves indicate wasted effort.

9. **SWIM DOWNHILL.** Lean on your chest until your hips and legs feel light.

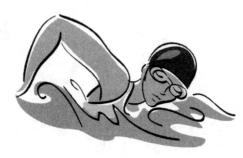

CHAPTER SEVEN:

PYRAMIDS
WHICH ONE DO YOU PREFER?

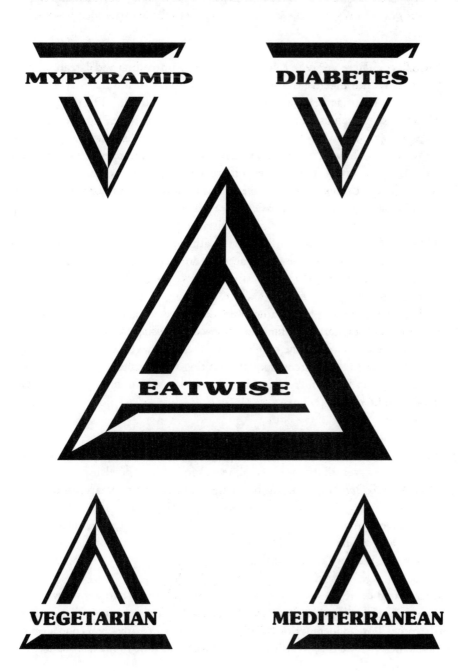

FOOD PYRAMIDS: WHICH ONE?

TWENTY WORDS OF NUTRITIONAL WISDOM

Eat a balanced diet, low in fat and sugar, high in fruits, vegetables, fiber and water and NEVER skip breakfast. — Don Alsbro Ed.D

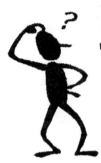

There are many books written on nutrition, and I realized that the objective of this book was not to try to summarize everything that has been written in the field, but to simplify the basics as much as possible.

Those of us who have been in the field of exercise and nutrition for many years have seen different philosophies, sometimes in direct conflict with each other. For example, in the field of exercise in the fifties and sixties, most athletes were discouraged from lifting weights because of the mistaken belief that increased muscle size would create muscle bound athletes who were unable to perform quick movements. Athletes were encouraged to do ballistic (bouncing) stretches as opposed to static stretches.

Athletes in training during hot weather were counseled to take salt tablets and stay away from the drinking fountain for fear of the water causing cramps. Often football coaches gave extra laps for anyone caught taking their helmet off during drills in high temperature. Women were discouraged from lifting weights because it was believed they would develop large, bulky muscles. We now know that all of the above have been proven to be myths.

The same is true for nutrition. One time we heard that sodium is bad for everyone, then we were told that it is okay for some people. We used to believe that if you ate three meals a day, you didn't need to take vitamins. We stopped using butter and switched to margarine only to learn that margarine with its trans fats can be as bad or worse than butter. Then we read one study claiming that coffee increases your chances of cancer, and then many other studies show that modest amounts of coffee are harmless and can be beneficial. We used to stress that dinner should be the largest meal of the day. We now know that these are all falsehoods.

Nutritional studies are like the Texas Two Step dance. You take two steps forward and one step back. However, when you look at the big picture you can see that gradually there becomes a preponderance of scientific evidence that clearly favors one idea over another. When you see this overwhelming evidence, it is time to make a change.

NEW DIETARY GUIDELINES FOR AMERICANS

Finding Your Way To a Healthier You   www.healthierus.gov/dietaryguidelines

In January 2005, the US Dept of Agriculture and US Dept of Health and Human Services released "Dietary Guidelines For Americans 2005." In all there were 23 general recommendations and 18 suggestions for older people, children and other specified populations. Some of the key guidelines are:

- Control weight through controlling calorie intake and engaging in 60 to 90 minutes of physical activity on most days of the week.
  NOTE: This is what this book has been all about—EAT LESS and EXERCISE MORE. If only we could learn this simple message!

- Consume two cups of fruit and 2.5 cups of vegetables a day (for a 2,000 calorie reference diet).

- Focus on whole-grain sources of grains. In general, at least half of the grains should come from whole grains.

- Consume three cups per day of fat-free or low fat milk or equivalent milk products.

- Choose a variety of fruits and vegetables each day. Select from all five vegetable sub groups (dark green, orange, legumes, starchy vegetables) several times a week.

- When selecting meat, poultry, dry beans, milk or milk products, make choices that are lean, low-fat or fat free.

- Consume less than 10% of calories from saturated fatty acids

- Keep total fat intake between 20-35% of calories with most fats coming from polyunsaturated and monounsaturated fats.

- Keep trans fatty acid consumption as low as possible.

- Choose fiber-rich fruits, vegetables and whole grains as often as possible

- Consume less than 2,300 mg (1 tsp of salt) of sodium per day

- Choose and prepare foods and beverages with little added sugars

- If you drink alcohol, keep it to one drink a day for women and two for men

ACTIVITY

- To REDUCE chronic adulthood disease EVERYONE should engage in at least 30 minutes of moderate physical activity, ABOVE the usual activity level, MOST days of the week.

- To MAINTAIN body weight and prevent gradual body weight gain, participate in at least 60 minutes of moderate physical activity MOST days of the week.

- To SUSTAIN weight LOSS, participate in at least 60-90 minutes of moderate activity, most days of the week, WHILE NOT exceeding caloric intake

CALORIC RECOMMENDATIONS BASED ON LIFESTYLE

	ACTIVITY	CALORIES
30 year old male	>30 min	2400
	30-60 min	2600
	<60 min	3000
30 year old female	>30 min	1800
	30-60 min	2000
	<60 min	2400

Basically, it is good to use these new guidelines. No longer are we trying to make our guidelines into "one size fits all." As the late heart doctor and marathon runner, George Sheehan used to say, "We are all an experiment of one." This is the first time that the government has added an exercise recommendation. Also, it gives people a lot of flexibility in planning their diets around their specific likes and dislikes.

MyPyramid

The U.S. Dept of Agriculture and the U.S. Dept of Health and Human Services have combined to produce a new symbol and interactive food guidance system that replaces the 1992 Food Guide Pyramid. It improves on the often criticized Food Guide Pyramid by emphasizing physical activity, whole grains, moderation in calories, a variety of foods and perhaps the biggest change of all—individualization.

MyPyramid allows individuals to personalize their approach by choosing a healthier lifestyle that balances nutrition and exercise. The new symbol was designed to be simple. Each colored strip on the pyramid is a sliver of the total diet. Orange represents grains, green is for vegetables, red for fruits, yellow means oils, blue represents dairy products and purple stands for meat and beans. On one side of the pyramid is a person climbing steps to remind consumers of the importance of daily physical activity.

Moderation is shown through the narrowing of each food group from bottom to top. The different widths of the food group bands represents proportionality. Widths suggest how much food a person should choose from each group, but are just a general guide. For example, the orange and green are the largest bands and the smallest band is the yellow band. For further personalization, individuals can visit the Web site at www.mypyramid.gov to see what kinds and amounts of food they should eat every day according to their age, gender and daily activity level.

MyPyramid website offers 12 individual nutrition plans based on gender, age and activity level. The site also offers sample menus, tips on making gradual dietary and exercise habits and detailed information on the various food groups. In the past, this level of personalized nutrition information was difficult to obtain short of meeting with a registered dietitian (RD).

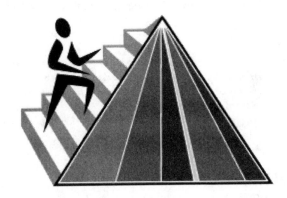

FRENCH WAY OF "DIETING"

1. Eat three meals a day
2. Keep portions small
3. Use lots of seasonal fruits and vegetables
4. Drink plenty of water
5. Savor wine
6. Walk everywhere
7. Allow yourself treats every once in a while
   French Women Don't Get Fat by Mireille Guiliano

FLEXITARIAN: *An "almost" vegetarian. Someone who generally prefers vegetables, fruits, low fat or no fat dairy products, whole grains and occasionally fish and poultry.*

OLDWAYS FOOD PYRAMIDS

"Nothing will benefit human health and increase the chances of survival of life on earth as much as the evolution to a vegetarian diet." — Albert Einstein

An interesting development over the past few years has been the introduction of food pyramids by Oldways Preservation and Exchange Trust of Boston. Oldways is a non-profit educational organization that promotes alternatives to the unhealthy foods that characterize eating patterns in industrialized countries. As a consequence, since 1993, Oldways has created four healthy dietary pyramids: Mediterranean, Asian, Latin American and Vegetarian. (www.oldwayspt.org)

One very vocal critic of the USDA Food Guides has been Dr. Neil Barnard, president of the Physicians Committee for Responsible Medicine (PCRM). The PCRM has successfully pushed for the inclusion of vegetarian diets in the federal guidelines.

Dr. Bernard states:

As a physician, it distresses me to no end to see patients that come as a result of the dangerous effects of a diet heavy on meat, fats, eggs and dairy products. We know a better way. Dietary changes should be the first line of treatment for heart disease, diabetes, hypertension, and many other diseases. It is clear to many … that the easiest way to stay slim and lower the risk for serious diseases is by eating a diet rich in plant food.

VEGETARIANISM

The Vegetarian Diet differs form the USDA Food Guide in many ways. Besides omitting meat, fish and poultry as primary sources of protein, it substitutes protein from soy, legumes, nuts, and seeds. Other differences are the emphasis on whole grains, plant oils, soy and rice milk.

Vegetarianism is divided into three major groups: vegan, lacto-ovo, and pesco. The vegans (pronounced vee-gan) abstain from eating all animal products, including milk, cheese, and eggs. The lacto-ovo vegetarians eat no flesh, but do eat eggs and dairy products, and the pesco-vegetarians eat dairy products, eggs, and fish, but no other animal flesh.

Of the three groups, the lacto-ovo vegetarians are the largest. Vegetarianism is one of the fastest growing lifestyles in the country. While each person has their own reasons for being vegetarian, for most, the main reason is better health.

> *VEGETARIAN TIMES. If you're seeking more information on the vegetarian lifestyle, an excellent source is Vegetarian Times, a monthly publication. www. vegetariantimes.com (877-717-8923).*

Health Benefits of Vegetarianism

All things considered, I think most nutritionists would agree that the healthiest diet is a plant based diet. The following are just a few of the many benefits of vegetarianism:

- **GREATER LONGEVITY** — Studies have consistently shown that vegetarians live longer, and their QUALITY of life while they're living is better.

- **FEWER HEART ATTACKS** — According to the American Medical Association a total vegetarian diet can prevent up to 90% of strokes and 97% of heart attacks.

- **FEWER WEIGHT PROBLEMS** — Vegetarians, generally, are not overweight.

- **LOWER CHOLESTEROL** — A plant based diet will usually result in cholesterol levels below 150.

- **LOWER BLOOD PRESSURE** — A simple vegetarian lifestyle change can reverse high blood pressure in a matter of weeks without drugs.

- **LESS DIABETES** — A plant based, low fat, high fiber diet in most situations can bring the blood sugar back to normal.

- **FEWER HEALTH PROBLEMS** — Lifestyle changes can help reduce occurrence of hemorrhoids, gallstones, kidney diseases, and diverticular diseases.

- **LESS CANCER** — These simple changes can prevent breast, prostate, and colon cancer.

THE LAST AND MOST IMPORTANT REASON:
IMPROVED QUALITY OF LIFE!

As Dr. Hans Diehl says,
"Health is not everything, but without it, everything is nothing."

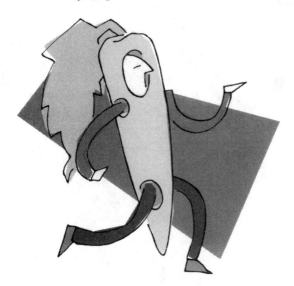

MEDITERRANEAN PYRAMID

The Mediterranean Diet has been called a compromise between the USDA Food Guide and the Vegetarian Diet. The addition of minimal amounts of meat, fish, poultry, and dairy products and the emphasis on olive oil and wine (not beer) has attracted many advocates. The diet gets most of its carbohydrates from fruits and vegetables, 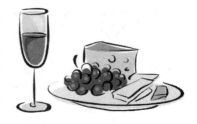 with the rest from breads, pastas and rice, and at least half of the fat content from monounsaturated oils such as olive oil. Milk is acceptable, but only skim or 1%.

THE EATWISE PYRAMID: A WIN, WIN PYRAMID

I originally intended to present what I consider to be the three "healthy" pyramids, i.e. Dr. Willett's Revised USDA pyramid, the Mediterranean and Vegetarian and let you pick and choose what you can live with for the rest of your life! However, as I was preparing this chapter on nutrition, I received a flyer from Oldways Preservation Trust with a new and different eating guide. It is exactly what I was looking for, i.e. a synthesis of the pyramids.

The EatWise Pyramid was developed by distinguished scientists from around the world. It emphasizes a balance among fats, proteins and carbohydrates. It stresses minimally processed carbohydrate foods like whole grains and cereals, vegetables, nuts, seeds, and fruit. It stresses plant oils like olive, canola and soy oil. These have high levels of unsaturated fats and low levels of saturated fats. It limits red meat to once or twice a week, and instead stresses protein from non-animal foods such as beans, nuts, seeds, whole grains, breads, and cereals. It limits highly processed carbohydrates like white flour and sugar and the saturated and trans fats found in pastries, donuts, and other processed foods. It also emphasizes moderate use of alcohol, exercise, and water.

"Eating right" should not mean "eating dull!" Eating the same foods, day in and day out-even if they're wholesome foods that provide a good mix of nutrients-can get "dull". Variety is the spice of life, and there is no reason you can't have variety, while still eating healthy. I'm a firm believer that our Maker didn't create "bad" food. However, he gave us the intelligence to make responsible choices.

What I like about the EatWise Pyramid is that you have a variety of foods that you can choose from. It uses practical, down-to-earth and realistic advice to map the route for individuals and families to turn away from poor eating and lifestyle habits. In addition to the EatWise Pyramid, Oldways has developed the Wise Eater's Plate and the EatWise Calorie Thermometer. For more information go to www. oldwayspt.org or call 617-896-4876.

The EatWise Pyramid

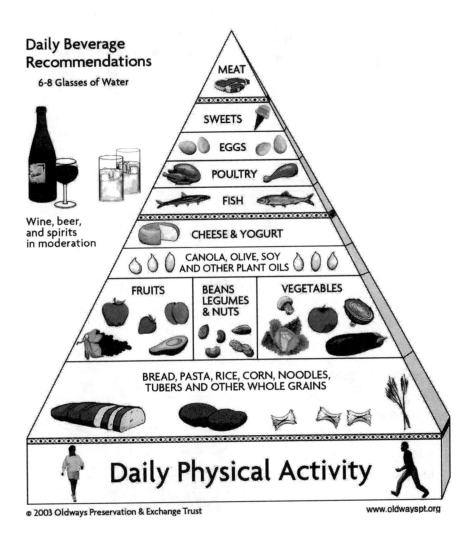

Reprinted with permission of Oldways Preservation Trust

Eat Fewer Fried Foods

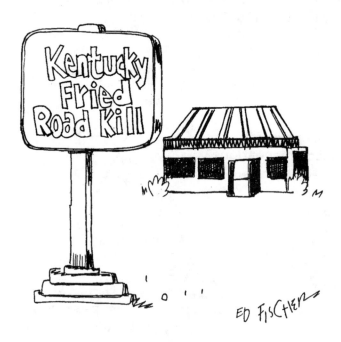

ED FISCHER

...Better Yet, Bake, Broil or Steam Foods

Feel less sluggish. Dry-fry your food in non-stick pans without oil or butter. Lightly steam or microwave vegetables instead of boiling them to save nutrients.

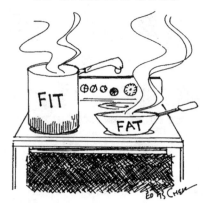

CHAPTER EIGHT:
DIETARY RULES
FOR A HEALTHY LIFE

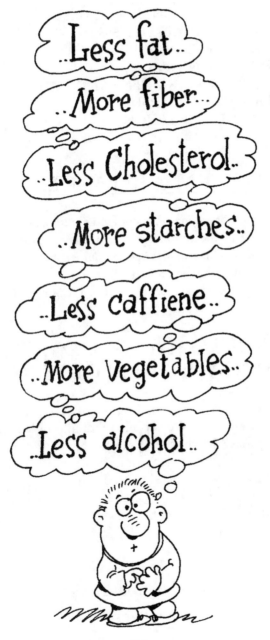

12 DIETARY RULES FOR A HEALTHY LIFE

1. EAT A BALANCED DIET.
2. CHOOSE "GOOD" FATS AND "GOOD" CARBOHYDRATES.
3. EAT PLENTY OF FRUITS AND VEGETABLES.
4. CAN YOU LIVE WITH THIS DIET?
5. INCREASE FIBER.
6. EAT BREAKFAST LIKE A KING OR A QUEEN.
7. CONSUME THE ULTIMATE FITNESS DRINK: WATER.
8. ACQUIRE LABEL READING SKILLS.
9. WATCH YOUR SERVING SIZES.
10. MAKE "GOOD" CHOICES WHEN EATING OUT.
11. SELECT TRAFFIC LIGHT FOODS.
12. CONSIDER SUPPLEMENTATION.

RULE 1: EAT A BALANCED DIET.

Each of the food pyramids emphasize major food groups. Each of these food groups provide some, but not all, the nutrients you need. You need food from all the groups to have a balanced diet. This rule was covered quite thoroughly in Chapter Seven. At the end of this chapter, after you've had a chance to look at all the diet guidelines, you will have the opportunity to prepare a diet you "can live with."

RULE 2: EAT "GOOD" FATS AND "GOOD" CARBOHYDRATES.

The notion that fat in general should be avoided was paramount in the 1992 USDA Food Guide. This stems from the observation that affluent Western countries have both high intakes of fat AND high rates of coronary heart disease. We now know that this correlation is only half-true. Societies in which people eat large portions of monounsaturated and polyunsaturated fat tend to have lower rates of heart disease. On the Greek island of Crete where fat constitutes 40% of the dietary calories (largely fish and olive oil), the rate of heart disease is much lower than Westernized nations with lower fat intake.

"Let Food Be Your Medicine."
— Hippocrates c. 400 BC

Unfortunately, in 1992 it was determined that it was too difficult to educate the American public about the differences in fats. Therefore, the USDA put out a clear, simple message: "Fat is bad." People accepted this message and the food industry started selling cookies, chips and other products that were low in fat but high in sweeteners such as high-fructose corn syrup.

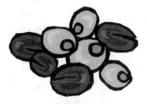

"GOOD" OR HEALTHY FATS: Monounsaturated fat (fat from avocados, olives and peanuts). Scientific studies indicate that these fats actually help lower total blood cholesterol levels. Polyunsaturated fat (found in vegetable oils and fish). These fats are thought by some nutrition experts to be neutral in raising or lowering blood cholesterol. Omega 3 fatty acids found in fish and some plant oils can reduce heart irregularities.

HEALTHY COOKING OILS: Fats are crucial to health. The trick is to know and eat the right kind. Almost every oil has saturated and unsaturated fats. Within the unsaturated there are two kinds, mono and poly. Within the poly, there are omega 3 and omega 6 fats. The omegas are known as essential fatty acids (EFAs), fats the body needs but can't produce on its own. These are easily obtained from fish products.

The health benefits of polyunsaturated fats are well documented. These benefits include significant cholesterol lowering effects and positive correlation to reducing heart disease. (Annals of Pharmacotherapy) Monounsaturated fats also show these same benefits. (New England Journal of Medicine) The best oils to use that

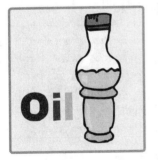

contain the highest amounts of monounsaturated and polyunsaturated fats are: Almond, flax, olive, and sesame oils.

"BAD" FATS: Saturated fats: These are found in all cheeses, whole milk and dairy products, meats and poultry. These fats are "bad" as they've been linked to heart disease, clogged arteries, weight gain, and breast and colon cancer.

"EXTRA BAD" FATS: Hydrogenated or Trans fats: These are truly the "bad" fats. They are found in nearly all processed foods and most fried foods.

HYDROGENATED OR TRANS FATS: Trans fat is a relatively new term to the nutrition vocabulary. The American public has gotten the message that saturated fats are bad for our health, but in the meantime, some sneaky food manufacturers have added a worse ingredient into our diet: trans fats. By using trans fats they can make the claim "no cholesterol" or "low in saturated fat," even though we have discovered that trans fats not only raises the LDL (bad) cholesterol, the same as saturated fats, but trans fats also reduce the HDL (good) cholesterol and raises the triglycerides, something saturated fat doesn't do. Trans fats are truly the "bad" guys in the fat arsenal. AVOID THEM.

These are fats that do not occur naturally but are created in a process called "partial hydrogenation." Partial hydrogenation is adding hydrogen gas to corn, soybean, and other saturated oils to make them more solid. The addition of hydrogen causes the oil to get harder, which allows the cookies or crackers to turn out properly and have longer shelf life. The problem is that the product has become "hydrogenated" with health properties worse than saturated fats.

WARNING: TAKE A CLOSE LOOK AT THE INGREDIENTS. IF YOU SEE THE WORDS "HYDROGENATED" OR "PARTIALLY HYDROGENATED" OILS AS ONE OF THE PRIMARY INGREDIENTS, BEWARE!

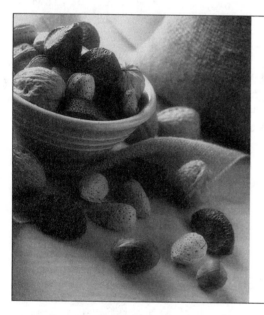

NUTS: Good or Bad?

Nuts contain fat. Therefore, many people question their place in a healthy eating plan. Most of the fat in nuts is monounsaturated and polyunsaturated fat rather than saturated. The fat composition of nuts is similar to that of olive oil. A 30 gram serving of mixed nuts contains 15 grams of total fat, but only 3 grams of saturated fat. In addition, they are a great source of protein & other nutritional goodies.

WHAT'S A SERVING?
A 1-ounce serving of nuts is approximately: 12 Macadamia nuts; 22 Almonds; 18 Cashews; 14 Walnut halves; 15 Pecan halves; 8 Brazil nuts; 12 Hazelnuts; 35 Peanuts; or 47 Pistachios. 1-ounce = 160-200 calories.

QUESTION:
HOW MUCH FAT IS HEALTHY?

According to an USDA survey, the average American consumes too many unhealthy fats (saturated and trans-fats) from meat, dairy products, desserts, and snack foods like cake, crackers, cookies, and doughnuts.

The new moderate-fat diet recommends eating more healthy fats (unsaturated and polyunsaturated) like olive oil, nuts, seeds, and fatty fish like salmon.

Which Diet Do You Follow?

AVERAGE AMERICAN DIET (High Fat Diet) *40% calories from fat (66 g.)**	**MODERATE - FAT DIET** *35% calories from fat (59 g.)**
Where's the fat? Beef, margarine, salad dressing, cheese, snacks and desserts	*Where's the fat?* Healthy, low-fat diet sources plus fatty fish, nuts, seeds, and healthy fats/oils
HEALTHY LOW-FAT DIET *20-30% calories from fat (35-50 g.)**	**ULTRA-LOW-FAT DIET** (CHIP, Ornish and Pritikin diets) *10-20% calories from fat (20-35 g.)**
Where's the fat? Fish, skinless poultry, lean meat, low-fat dairy, and small amounts of healthy fats/oils	*Where's the fat?* Fish, skinless poultry, and small amounts of healthy oil **Based on a 1500 calorie diet.*

BOTTOM LINE: When making a choice of fats, opt for mono or poly unsaturated fats. But remember: Fat is fat, is fat, is fat, is fat... IN OTHER WORDS, LESS STEAK AND MORE FISH!

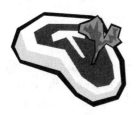
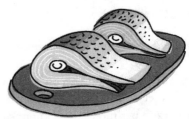

STEAK ON A 10% FAT DIET

HIGH FAT	LOW FAT
Breakfast	

Granola	Raisin Bran
Toast with Butter	Toast with no butter
Lots of Jelly	1 tsp. of jelly
Whole Milk	Skim Milk
680 Cal. 28 fat grams	**406 Cal. 2 fat grams**
252 fat cal. (37% fat)	*18 fat cal (14% fat)*

Lunch

Tuna (packed in oil)	Tuna (packed in water)
Lots of mayonnaise	Low fat mayonnaise
Coke	Diet Coke
Potato Chips	Plate of fresh fruit
830 Cal. 47 fat grams	**360 Cal. 6 fat grams**
423 fat cal. (51% fat)	*36 fat cal. (10% fat)*

Dinner

Porterhouse steak	London Broil
Baked Potato with everything	Baked Potato with low-fat toppings
Salad with Blue-cheese dressing	Salad with fat-free ranch dressing
Glass of Wine	Water or Coffee
1,588 Cal. 111 fat grams	**787 Cal. 9 fat grams**
999 fat cal (63% fat)	*81 fat cal (10% fat)*

Totals

Total fat calories: 1,674	Total fat calories: 135
Total calories: 3,098	Total calories: 1,553
% of Fat: 54%	% of Fat: 9%

*Slide from the Nutri-graphics slide presentation by Eve Lowrey

If you were to consume this high-fat diet on a daily basis, the difference between the high-fat diet of 3098 calories and the low-fat diet of 1553 calories equals 46, 350 calories extra per month or 13 pounds per month, 156 pounds per year!

CARBOHYDRATES: What are Carbohydrates? They are the primary energy-providing nutrient for the muscles and brain. Carbohydrates should be at least 60% of your daily caloric intake. In general, there are two forms:

Complex Carbohydrates - Long lasting energy: Grains, Bread, Cereals, Rice, Pasta, Potatoes, Peas, Corn, Legumes.

Simple Carbohydrates - Quick energy, but shorter duration: Fruits, Sugars, and most Candies.

Carbohydrates are contained in a vast array of foods, everything from the most virtuous vegetable to the most decadent treat. All carbohydrates contain sugars. However, these sugars exist in different forms and by different names.

SUGAR HAS MANY NAMES

In general, the difference between carbohydrates is the rate at which they enter the bloodstream as glucose or energy. The more sugar there is, and the faster it is released. This quicker release will result in the sugar "rush." We have all experienced this around 10 a.m. or 4 p.m. after we've had that candy bar, or doughnut.

In the digestion process, the speed of digestion of the sugar molecule is dependent upon whether the carbohydrate is a simple one, meaning that it is not encumbered by other substances in the food such as fiber or fat, or if it's a complex carb that will take longer to enter the small intestine as energy. For example, a milk chocolate bar gives up its energy much quicker than an apple or whole grain oatmeal.

Sugar calories when not encumbered by other substances are sometimes called "simple" carbohydrates. These are referred to as "empty" calories, for they provide very little nutrients and vitamins, little lasting energy, and contribute to weight gain. These sugars are commonly found in candy, cookies, soft drinks, and table sugar. Sugar consumption per capita in the U.S. has risen from 40 lbs. in the 1950's to almost 150 lbs. in 2000.

> ### SUGAR HAS MANY NAMES:
>
> *Sugar appears on labels under many names: sucrose, glucose, dextrose, sorbitol, fructose, maltose, fructose, molasses, and maple syrup.*
> *READ THE LABEL.*
> *A food is likely to be high in sugar if its ingredient list shows one of the above first or second, or if it shows several of them.*

They are referred to as "simple" calories because as soon as they enter the system they are converted to glucose or energy. This produces a sugar "high" which is followed by a sugar "low" when the insulin arrives to take the glucose away. For diabetics this insulin doesn't arrive.

One teaspoon of sugar contains 16 calories.

DID YOU KNOW:

THIS PRODUCT...		CONTAINS THIS MUCH SUGAR?
12 oz soft drink (128-160 cal.)	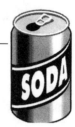	**8-10 tsp.**
8 oz. Kool Aid (96 cal.)	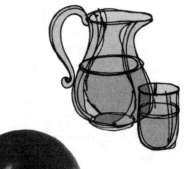	**6 tsp.**
1 Doughnut (96 cal.)		**6 tsp.**
		KRISPY KREME GLAZED DONUT: 200 calories, 110 cal. fat (55%)
1 Cupcake (96 cal.)	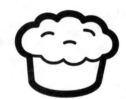	**6 tsp.**
2 oz chocolate bar (96-128 cal.)	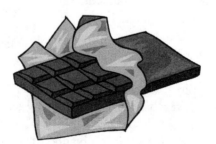	**6-8 tsp.**

Since most nutritionists feel that carbohydrates should be our main dietary source, it is important to spend extra time discussing them. In my previous book "The Best Little Book of Wellness," I had two dietary rules: Increase your consumption of complex carbohydrates and decrease your consumption of simple carbohydrates. In general, that is still good advice, but like fats, it needs to be expanded upon.

Carbohydrates occur in three forms, depending on the number of saccharide (sugar) units that make up the molecule. Mono and disaccharides are called simple sugars, whereas polysaccharides are referred to as complex sugars or starches

Simple sugars are known as glucose, fructose, dextrose, sucrose and lactose. More than 100 substances called sugars exist. They are found in soft drinks, desserts, many cereals, and canned foods. The average American consumes 150 pounds of sugars and sweeteners per year.

Poly-sugars are found primarily in vegetables, fruits, and grains. Although fruits are high in natural sugars, they are also high in vitamins, minerals, protein, fiber and water. Thus, they don't enter the bloodstream as fast as the simple sugars, so there is less need for insulin. Simply put, with poly-sugars we don't have sugar "highs" and "lows."

For the purpose of this book, we need to be aware that, like fats, trying to divide carbohydrates into simple (bad) and complex (good) is too simplistic. Not all simple carbohydrates are bad, and not all complex carbohydrates are good.

LOW-CARB DIETS

CONCEPT: Refined carbohydrates found in white flour, white rice and sugary treats, cause blood sugar or glucose to rise. High glucose, in turn, prompts the body to churn out large amounts of insulin, the stuff that shoves glucose into the body's cells so it can be burned for energy. By drastically cutting carbohydrates, a "low carb" diet reduces glucose and insulin, and many scientists believe the risks of heart disease, diabetes and obesity.

GLYCEMIC INDEX

In the 1990's there was extensive research into the effects of carbohydrates on the blood sugar. This is called the glycemic index. The glycemic index is a measure of how carbohydrate-containing foods affect blood glucose levels. You might expect foods with more simple sugars, such as candy and soft drinks, to have higher glycemic indices than baked potatoes and corn flakes. But that's not always the case. Baked potatoes and corn flakes actually have higher glycemic indices than jellybeans and pop.

Many of the "low carb" diets utilize the glycemic index. Its role in obesity is debated by researchers and nutritionists. They argue that the glycemic index has not been proven to be beneficial for weight loss. Also, it unfairly penalizes some healthy foods (mainly fruits and plant based carbohydrates), and confuses dieters.

The potato in particular has taken an unfair hit. A medium baked potato (minus the toppings) is only 100 calories, and provides 45% of the daily value for Vitamin C, 21% of the daily value for potassium, no fat, and is rich in fiber. The same could be said for the carbohydrates in brown rice, whole wheat pasta, and other whole wheat products.

Some nutritionists feel that a more realistic approach to use – instead of the glycemic index (GI) – is the glycemic load (GL), which is an estimate of both the quality AND the quantity of carbohydrates in the diet (the glycemic index gives only quality). Therefore, the GL measures two factors: the amount of carbohydrates in the meal and the nature (GI value) of that carbohydrate. Advocates believe that if you use the GL correctly you can eat smaller portions of high GI foods.

My good friend, Ronda Gates, MS, who has degrees in pharmacy and nutrition and has been delivering health programs since 1978, says, "Instead of putting emphasis on the glycemic index, focus on the more sensible glycemic load – the index that combines glycemic index and food serving size." To receive Ronda's educational Lifestyle newsletters, e-mail ronda@rondagates.com.

> *"People seem to have forgotten that it is the calories that count and exercise that matters when it comes to weight loss."*
>
> — Judi Adams, Dietitian

George Blackburn, associate director of nutrition at Harvard Medical School, says that we should look at the entire meal, instead of individual items. "When you combine fruits, vegetables, low fat dairy, and a variety of plant-based carbohydrates, you end up with a low, glycemic index-load meal." (USA Today D-2)

Judi Adams, a registered dietitian and president of the "Wheat Foods Council," is fed up with the glycemic debate. She says, "It's stupid to even consider the glycemic index. There are no long term studies that show the glycemic index makes any difference in obesity or diabetes. People seem to have forgotten that it is the calories that count and exercise that matters when it comes to weight loss." She goes on to say that, "Most of the world bases their diets on carbohydrates and they don't have the obesity rates we do because they eat less and exercise more." (USA Today D-2)

Dan Gifford, president of Oldways Preservation Trust and developer of the "Eatwise Pyramid," says, " High carb diets have worked well for centuries in other countries, but people in the U.S. have trampled carbs because this is a "hula hoop" society with a "quick fix" mentality."

I'm sure we will hear much more on this subject, but hopefully common sense will prevail. The research seems to indicate that while the low carb diet works better initially, that over the long haul, it is no more successful, and in many cases less successful than the diet that encourages intake of complex carbohydrates.

> *Researchers from Stanford University and Yale University analyzed 107 low-carb diets and concluded that weight loss was because the diet contained fewer calories, not through restricting carbs. — American Medical Journal (April 9, 2003)*

My thoughts on the subject are that our Creator didn't create junk food, man did! It makes more sense to eat a plant based diet, with smaller amounts of red meat, poultry, and fish, AND move the body!

ALMOND JOY

According to a study reported in the Journal of Obesity, scientists at Loma Linda University compared two low-calorie diets that were similar in calorie and protein intake, but varied in fat and carbohydrates. The higher fat diet was composed of 39% fat (majority coming from 84 g. of almonds) and 32% carbohydrates. The higher carbohydrate diet had 18% fat and 53% carbohydrates (from complex carbohydrate sources). After 24 weeks, those on the almond supplemented (fat) diet lost 62% more weight, 56% more body fat, and 50% more of their waist than those on the complex carbohydrate diet.

MORAL: Don't be afraid to eat healthy fats (nuts, seeds, olives and fatty fish). Just be sure they replace (not in addition to) the calories from carbohydrates.

GLYCEMIC FOODS

The foods listed below are indexed according to their ability to raise blood glucose after eating.

GREEN LIGHT	**YELLOW LIGHT**	**RED LIGHT**
Low: Digested Slowly	*Moderate*	*High: Digested Quickly*
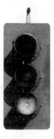	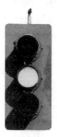	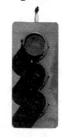

GREEN LIGHT	YELLOW LIGHT	RED LIGHT
Beans	Whole grain breads	Potatoes
Nuts	Brown rice	White bread
Seeds	Old fashioned oatmeal	White rice
Most fruits	Whole wheat pasta	Sugar products
Most vegetables	Whole grain cereals	Baked goods
Air popped popcorn		White flour products
		(cookies, cakes, candy)

Basic Rule:

CHOOSE whole grain products.
RELY ON fruits, legumes, and vegetables.
AVOID simple sugar products (sucrose, glucose, fructose, etc.)

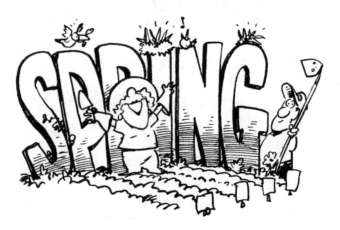

CARBOHYDRATES, WHOLE GRAINS, FRUITS AND VEGETABLES

Carbohydrates are readily available low calorie sources of energy. Besides providing us with an efficient source of energy, they assure the vitamins and minerals needed for good health and fiber that is essential for proper digestion. Compared to proteins and fat, they are digested more quickly. However, like proteins and fat, if you eat too many and are not exercising, they will be stored as fat. Up to 60% of the calories you eat should come from this group of foods. Complex carbohydrates have lots of vitamins and minerals and include fresh fruits and vegetables, whole grains, beans, and brown rice.

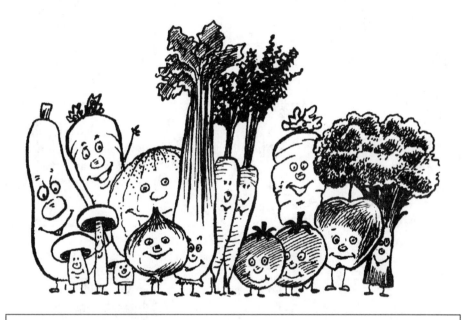

Up to 60% of the calories you eat should come from "complex carbohydrates"

BOTTOM LINE: As a general rule, try to obtain your carbohydrates from a plant-based diet of fruits and vegetables and avoid to a large extent the refined sugars found in candy bars, white bread, pastries, soft drinks, syrups and jams, potatoes, ready-to-eat cereals, and whole milk, especially if you are overweight or have a tendency toward diabetes. Again, as it has been stressed throughout this book, you are responsible for your destiny. While the gun may be loaded (genetics), you determine by your lifestyle choices whether the trigger is pulled.

The following one-day menu, shows that the selection of the proper amounts and kinds of food provides a considerable amount of nutrition for people losing weight. For women, 1200 calories are the minimum recommended number of calories per day, and for men, 1500 calories are the minimum recommended amount.

SAMPLE MENU

1200 CALORIES	1500 CALORIES	
BREAKFAST		
1 c.	1 c.	multi-grain cereal
.5 c.	.5 c.	low fat milk
5	1	banana
MORNING SNACK		
3	5	crackers
1 Tbs.	1 Tbs.	low-sugar jam
LUNCH		
1 oz.	2 oz.	turkey
.25	.25	avocado, lettuce, tomato
0	2 tsp.	low calorie mayonnaise
2 slice	2 slice	whole wheat bread
.5 c.	1 c.	grapes
MID-AFTERNOON SNACK		
2	4	fig bars
DINNER		
3 oz.	3 oz.	grilled halibut
2 tsp.	3 tsp.	low cal margarine
1 tsp.	1 tsp.	lemon juice
1.5 c.	1.5 c.	peas and mushrooms
1	1	dinner roll
1 tsp.	2 tsp.	low cal margarine
SNACK		
0	50	unsalted pretzels (sticks)
TOTALS		
25% Fat	17% Fat	
57% Carbohydrate	65% Carbohydrate	
18% Protein	18% Protein	

RULE 3. EAT PLENTY OF FRUITS
AND VEGETABLES

Most of us can recall our mothers telling us to eat up the spinach, broccoli or whatever was still on our plate because it was "good" for us. As usual, our mothers were right. A diet rich in fruits AND vegetables can:

• Decrease the chances of heart disease.
• Protect against many cancers.
• Help us avoid diverticular disease which can lead to the painful diverticulitis.
• Lower blood pressure.
• Protect against the eye diseases of cataracts and macular degeneration.
• Be a dietary source of calcium to protect against osteoporosis.
• Provide a variety in our diet.

In 1991 the National Cancer Institute instituted a "5 - A - Day," urging us to get five servings a day of fruits and vegetables. This has since been endorsed by the USDA, World Health Organization, American Heart Assoc., and many others. The average American gets less than four servings a day and that includes French fries, which, unfortunately, is one of our most popular eating choices. Numerous studies show that you do not get the same health benefits from potatoes that you do from the other fruits and vegetables.

A recent study of the fruit and vegetable intake of our children and adolescents from the ages of 2 to 18 found that only 20% of them were getting at least three servings and 25% of these servings were in the form of French fries. Having analyzed hundreds of diets of college students, I can substantiate this finding. In my healthful living class, they were required to analyze their diets, and it was rare to find a student who had over 15 grams of fiber and 3 servings of fruits and vegetables per day.

Three quarters of your plate should be taken up by fruits and vegetables and you should strive to make your plate as colorful as you can. Make your plate full of bold colors such as the red tomato, the orange sweet potato, green peas and beans, yellow corn, juicy blueberries and red strawberries, the green spinach and broccoli, orange slices, yellow squash, orange carrots, the orange cantaloupe, red, green, and yellow peppers, and deep red lettuce. These colorful fruits and vegetables contain the phytonutrients necessary to protect against cancer and other diseases.

Five a day is a start, but it is often loosely interpreted. For example, two glasses of orange juice for breakfast, an apple and French fries for lunch, and a baked potato for dinner meet the target of five, but these would not be considered quality calories (with the exception of the apple). Aim for 7-9 servings of fruits and vegetables. We are looking for quality, not quantity.

RULE 4: CAN YOU LIVE WITH THIS DIET ?

This is probably the most important rule. There are literally thousands of diets out there. You can't pick up a magazine without having at least one diet inside and they all promise that you will lose weight . We have the Grapefruit Diet, Ice Cream Diet, Peanut Butter Diet, Sugar Busters, Weight Watchers, Zone, and many more. Some of them are good, but most make outlandish claims with no research to back it up. Today I was reading a health magazine, and it featured the Starch Blocker Diet. This diet advocates taking a supplement made from white kidney beans that, according to the developers, causes 70 percent of the starch you eat to pass through your system undigested. According to the authors, you don't have to reduce calories so you don't get hungry. What a neat idea. I can eat as much as I want and not gain weight. Unfortunately, this diet is another one of many get-rich schemes that will make the authors a lot of money and leave a lot of disappointed people in its wake. This diet has no public scientific research on humans to back up the claims, and yet it has become a popular diet. The American public is always looking for the magic pill. There is no secret to weight loss, it's simply "eat right and exercise daily." So simple, but most people don't want to hear it.

The latest fad is to follow the high protein, low carbohydrate diets. These diets, ban all carbohydrates, and encourage high protein consumption and unlimited saturated fats, especially red meat, butter, eggs, and cheese.

> *Despite the hype about low carb diets, the research continues to bear long held beliefs that in the long term, it's a balanced and varied, lower in fat and sugar (especially added fat and sugar), high in fiber, calorie sufficient diet that sets the stage for living an active long as possible life. Chicken is a wiser choice than "red meat" and fish is a better choice than chicken. In fact, the closer you go to a plant based diet the better chance you have to avoid the silent progression of diseases that can kill you-especially if exercise and healthy fueling of this fabulous human machinery are ignored!* — Ronda Gates, MS, CLC
>
> *"Smart Lifestyles" e-mail newsletter, Feb. 2, 2004. (e-mail: ronda@rondagates.com)*

A diet like this is a short term solution to a long range problem. Sure if you follow the plan as prescribed, you will lose about 5-10 lbs in the first two weeks. However, that weight loss is primarily due to the water loss or dehydration produced by the foods consumed and by limiting calories. Preliminary data indicates that the "low-carb" participants eat about 1,800 calories a day. Anyone is bound to lose weight under those conditions, but the long-term results are no more impressive than any of the other diet plans. No one can, or should, continue eating large amounts of saturated fats and proteins if they want to avoid major health problems.

BOTTOM LINE: ANY DIET THAT PERMANENTLY ELIMINATES FRUITS AND/OR VEGETABLES SHOULD BE AVOIDED!

SHOULD I CONSIDER A HIGH PROTEIN DIET?

QUESTION: *"I have a friend who lost a lot of weight on the high protein diet. Is that a good diet for weight loss?"*

ANSWER: *"Many people have lost weight on the high protein diet. But the question is, 'Does the weight stay off?' Another good question is, 'What did she (he) actually lose?'"*

The high protein diet promotes a water and muscle loss. In the absence of essential carbohydrates from food, the muscle protein is broken down to produce glucose. Therefore, muscle mass is reduced. This works against long-term weight loss. The more muscle you have, the more calories you burn. Preserve your muscle mass by eating enough carbohydrates. The high protein diet also promotes dehydration. Water is necessary for protein to be metabolized. Some of the pounds lost on a high protein diet are water loss.

High protein diets are also risky. High protein diets are usually high in fat. Research continues to validate that high protein diets are related to coronary heart disease, diabetes, and increased risk of cancer. High protein diets cause the body to lose calcium which increases the risk of osteoporosis. High protein diets also cause stress on the kidneys, and, for women, high protein diets affect hormone levels and can complicate PMS and menopause symptoms.

Do yourself a favor. Choose a healthy eating program that includes foods as grown, the way food comes in nature. Abundant intake of vegetables, fruits, whole grain breads and cereals, and beans gives you essential vitamins, minerals, antioxidants, and phytochemicals. Doesn't it make sense to include a rich variety of these foods to reach and maintain your healthy weight and enjoy vibrant health?

Evelyn Cole Kissinger, MS, RD, IBCLC, Lifestyle Consultant / Registered Dietitian Nutritionist

PROTEIN

What is protein? Protein helps to build and repair muscle and organ tissue. While it is a good energy source, carbohydrates are better. Protein needs vary depending on the person's height, weight, and physical activity. Most individuals do not need to consume more than 6-8 ounces of protein per day, or no more than 20% of total calories. Excess protein passes through the body as urine, thus making you dehydrated.

ANIMAL SOURCES: All meats (also high fat), fish, poultry, dairy products, eggs.
VEGETABLE SOURCES: Beans (all varieties), nuts, peanut butter (also high fat), tofu, soy products.

How Much Protein Do I Need?

Contrary to popular belief, a little protein goes a long way. For a sedentary person the RDA for protein is about .4 gram per pound of body weight. This means 58 grams per day for an inactive 145 lb. woman. An active 145 lb. woman needs .5-.6 g. per pound. Thus, for an active woman that's about 73-87 g. per day. The difference between 58 g. and 73 g. is equivalent to 2 ounces or 17 g. of tuna.

RULE 5. INCREASE FIBER

(NOTE: This happens automatically when you increase complex carbohydrates)

FIBER HAS THE FOLLOWING BENEFITS:
- Relieves constipation by being a natural laxative.
- Helps control obesity by filling up the body with fewer calories.
- Helps prevent diverticulosis which sometimes leads to diverticulitis.
- Helps prevent hemorrhoids.
- Helps prevent colo-rectal cancer.
- Lowers blood cholesterol levels which is a major heart disease risk factor.
- Lowers the blood sugar levels by slowing down glucose metabolism.

There are two categories of fiber:

SOLUBLE (BINDERS): Found in fruits, vegetables, and grains. This type of fiber forms a gel as it is digested and then absorbs water in the intestinal tract increasing stool bulk. This gel also moderates blood sugar levels. Studies have shown that soluble fiber lowers the bad cholesterol (LDL) without decreasing the good cholesterol (HDL).

INSOLUBLE (SCRUBBERS): Found in woody stalks, peels, and skins of fruits and vegetables, and in the bran (seed coat) of whole grains. This type of fiber moves food more quickly through your digestive system, ushering out cancer causing substances and reducing the risk of colo-rectal cancer. With this fiber, the "transit" time can be as low as 14 hours, without it as much as 48-72 hours.

DAILY REQUIREMENT: While there is no established RDA for fiber, most authorities feel that the average person should try to consume 25-35 grams of fiber per day. In my college nutrition classes, it was rare to encounter a student with an intake higher than 15 grams. NOTE: If you're currently way below 25-25, don't try and increase it in one day, but make it a gradual process. According to Dr. Roizen in "RealAge," the average American consumes an average of 12 grams of fiber per day. Consuming a daily fiber diet of 25 grams can reduce arterial aging and make your RealAge as much as three years younger.

Eat More Fiber

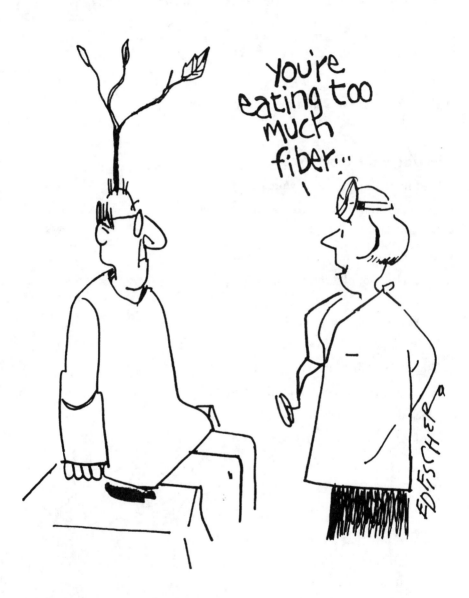

(Reprinted with permission from Dr. Jeff Haebig, Wellness Quest©)

HOW TO GET 40 GRAMS OF FIBER IN ONE DAY

Baked Potato .... 4 grams
Apple w/skin .... 4 grams
Whole grain cereal or Oatmeal .... 6-8 grams
Cantaloupe .... 4 grams
Beans (1 cup) .... 16 grams
Raisins (.5 cup) .... 6 grams

WARNING: Increase your fiber intake gradually.

Meeting your Fiber Needs

- Use brown rice instead of white rice.
- Choose fresh fruits over canned fruits or juices.
- Select whole grain breads.
- Leave the peels on fruits and vegetables.
- Eat a salad (with low fat or non fat dressing) every day.
- Use oats as a filler in casseroles or meat loaf.
- Eat beans and peas often.
- Use whole grain flours when you bake.
- Have a high fiber cereal or muffin daily.
- Snack on raw vegetables and fresh fruit.
- Eat foods in their natural states.

WARNING:
Drink plenty of liquids (water) to help minimize the bloating and gas that some people experience when they suddenly increase fiber in their diets.

WARNING:
Never sit close to the campfire when eating beans!

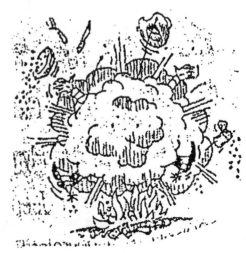

142

OATMEAL DELIGHT

Pre-mix in a large container:

		ANALYSIS (1 SERVING):
Rolled Old Fashioned Whole Grain Oats	5c. (32 oz)	83 calories
Oat Bran	2c. (8 oz)	3 g. fat
Wheat Germ	1c. (5 oz)	(22% >1 g. sat.)
Flax Seed (ground)	1c. (2 oz)	3 g. protein
Wheat Bran	1c. (2 oz)	13 g. carbs
		4 g. fiber

Place 3 cups of water on high heat. Add 1 cup of above mixture. Add 1 tsp. of vanilla extract and 1/2 tsp. of ground cinnamon. Add (any or all) if desired: 1 apple, sliced with skin; 1/4 cup of raisins; 1/2 cup of blueberries; 1/4 cup of almonds. After coming to a boil, cook on low heat for 15-20 minutes, stirring occasionally. NOTE: You could substitute unsweetened apple or white grape juice for the water. Makes 4 servings.

Above recipe was modified from an original recipe provided by LTC (Ret) Art Osborne of Columbus, GA

RULE 6. EAT BREAKFAST LIKE A KING OR A QUEEN

Our largest and most nutritious meal should be breakfast. It is a meal that we should NEVER skip. This is exactly the opposite of what we used to believe. If we did have breakfast, it would be a small one, i.e. coffee, juice, and a pop tart. Then we would have a moderate sized lunch, and this would be followed by a large supper which was designed to replace the calories that we'd expended during the day. We now believe that breakfast and supper should be reversed. We need to put "gasoline" or food in the body to start the day, especially since we've gone for 12-15 hours with no gas in the tank. The literal meaning of breakfast is "break the fast." Studies have shown that by eating a nutritious breakfast, you will jump start your metabolism by 17%, which is significant if you're trying to lose weight.

In a Vanderbilt study, overweight "breakfast skippers" who started eating breakfast, lost an average of 17 pounds in 12 weeks. What's more powerful, breakfast eaters were better able to maintain their weight loss than breakfast skippers.

Breakfast is an opportunity to get fiber and energy foods like whole grain cereals, fruit, and whole grain breads. We can get over 50% of our daily fiber requirement in breakfast. This gives us the energy to start the day. Then at lunch we can have a protein source such as turkey, tuna fish, chicken, or a Veggie sub, along with some carbohydrates in the form of fruits or vegetables and a cup of tea. Most nutritionists feel that up to 60% of our daily calories should be consumed by noon. Then at night we can have a light meal that is easily digested before we retire.

NUTRITIOUS BREAKFASTS

Here are some breakfasts that are low in calories, high fiber, high in vitamins and minerals and high in energy. ENJOY!

1. 1/2 grapefruit, low fat mozzarella cheese, and fresh tomato slices broiled on a whole grain English muffin.
2. Non-fat yogurt with fresh fruit, crumpet with a dab of honey, and skim milk.
3. Sliced banana, toasted bagel with natural peanut butter, skim milk.
4. Chilled fresh melon, assorted low fat cheeses, sour dough rye roll, skim milk.
5. Fresh strawberries, scrambled eggs (egg substitute), with salsa, English muffin.
6. Freshly squeezed grapefruit juice, hot or cold cereal with skim milk, whole wheat toast.
7. Freshly squeezed orange juice, homemade bran muffin, skim milk.
8. Baked apple, hot oatmeal with skim milk, whole wheat toast.

BREAKFAST SKIPPERS

A University of Massachusetts study found that people who skip breakfast entirely, are 4.5 times more likely to be obese than those who eat it regularly. Reason: Spreading out calories over the day keeps insulin levels more stable, thus reducing the storage of blood sugars.

TYPICAL AMERICAN BREAKFAST			HEALTHY BREAKFAST		
	Calories	Fat Calories		Calories	Fat Calories
Bacon, 3 Slices	110	81	Banana	81	0
Scrambled Eggs (3)	330	216	Oatmeal w/Blueberries & Nonfat Yogurt	320	27
Hash Browns, 1 cup	355	162	Whole Wheat Toast (2) w/Jam	140	18
Hot Chocolate w/milk	213	72	Orange Juice (8 oz.)	110	0
Orange Juice (8 oz.)	110	0	Hot Tea	0	0
Coffee w/sugar/cream	45	20			
TOTALS	1165	551 (47%)	TOTALS	651	45 (7%)

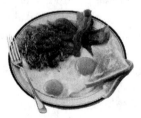

HEART-ATTACK ON A PLATE!

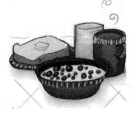

LIFE SAVING!

RULE 7. ULTIMATE FITNESS DRINK: WATER

Many people who are trying to lose weight avoid drinking water in the mistaken belief that it can promote weight gain because of water retention. This is false.

WATER SHOULD BE CONSIDERED A "MAGIC POTION" FOR THE FOLLOWING REASONS:

- Water suppresses the appetite naturally while aiding digestion.

- Insufficient water intake forces the liver to do some of the kidney's function. Water stimulates kidney activity, freeing the liver to metabolize fat.

- When the body gets less water, it perceives this as a threat to survival. The body holds onto every drop, resulting in swollen feet, legs, etc. Giving the body plenty of water helps fight the body's tendency for fluid retention.

- Water improves glandular function.

- Water helps to maintain proper muscle tone by helping them contract and prevents dehydration.

- Water helps rid the body of waste.

- Water can help prevent or relieve constipation.

- Proper hydration helps prevent heat exhaustion and heat stroke. Coffee is a diuretic and should never be used for fluid replacement. The same with pop. In the troop medical clinics during summer military training, we treated many soldiers for heat problems who thought that the morning coffee counted for water. We would ask the soldiers if they would consider putting coffee in their military vehicle's radiator, instead of water. The body needs pure water.

The average person should drink 8-10 eight ounce glasses of water every day. An overweight person needs one additional glass for every 25 lbs. of excess weight. This amount should be increased if you exercise briskly or if the weather is hot and dry. Many people are afraid of drinking water during a workout because they fear getting cramps. Actually, dehydration will give you cramps.

YOUR DAILY DRINKING REQUIREMENT

The old formula — everyone needs eight glasses of water a day — has been replaced by formulas based on gender and body weight.

Male Water Requirement:	Body Weight _____ X .35 =	_____ oz.
Female Water Requirement:	Body Weight _____ X .31 =	_____ oz.

Example: A 132 lb. woman needs to drink 41 oz of water a day (132 X .31) or five 8 oz. glasses. She'll get the rest of her daily water supply from food and metabolic processes.

More than 75 percent of our body is made up of water. When you don't drink enough, your blood doesn't flow properly, and the digestive track doesn't run smoothly. You typically lose 10 cups of water per day – 2 cups to sweating and evaporation, 2 cups to breathing, and 6 cups to waste removal. You can replace up to 2 cups through the water in the foods you eat, but you have to make up the remaining 8 cups by drinking fluids-water being the best choice.

> **THE AVERAGE PERSON SHOULD DRINK 8-10 EIGHT OUNCE GLASSES OF WATER EVERY DAY.**

Sport drinks like "Gatorade" are okay when you exercise for more than an hour, since they provide fluid as well as easily digestible energy. Water is sufficient and preferred for shorter workouts Many of the tennis players will cut the sport drink by adding 50% water and take this during their match.

Drink 6-8 glasses of purified water or unsweetened fruit or vegetable juice each day. Notice how keenly your mind and body function with adequate fluids.

... BUT NOT ALL AT BEDTIME!

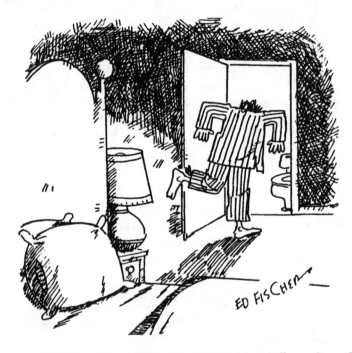

(Reprinted with permission from Dr. Jeff Haebig, Wellness Quest©)

SIGNS YOU'RE NOT DRINKING ENOUGH H2O:

Bad Breath • Pasty Mouth/Tongue • Dark Color/Smelly Urine
Intestinal Cramping • Difficult Bowels • Dry Skin • Headaches

RULE 8. ACQUIRE LABEL READING SKILLS

Nutrition labeling is the shopper's right to know the nutritional quality of the foods they're purchasing. The labels have a standard format, and once you understand the terms, reading the label is simple. Basic Rule: Label reading should be practiced by everyone who buys groceries.

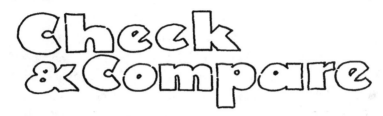

Here are some key items to look for:

- **Serving Size:**   Is your serving the same size as the one on the label? If you eat double the serving size listed, you need to double the nutrient and calorie values.

> **NOTE:** *A 20-oz. bottle of Coke, for instance, says 100 calories, but that's for 8 ounces (the bottle of soda actually has 250 calories). Similarly, the label on a muffin, frozen entrée, or even a small bag of chips may say two or three servings, so you have to double or triple the calories, grams of fat, and milligrams of sodium.*

- **Calories:**   How does this fit into your daily calorie allowance?

- **Dietary Fiber:**   This includes both soluble and insoluble fiber. Strive for a daily allowance of at least 25 grams of fiber.

- **Protein:**   Most Americans get more protein than they need. Where there is animal protein, there is also fat and cholesterol.

- **Vitamins & Minerals:**   Your goal is 100% of each for a day. Don't count on one food to do it all. The only ones required to be listed are Vitamins A and C, calcium and iron.

- **Total Fat:**   This is a key one. By limiting your calories from fat, you lower your risk for heart disease, cancer, and obesity.

Basic Rule: Label reading should be practiced
by everyone who buys groceries.

- **Saturated & Trans Fats:** All fat is not equal. Saturated fat is a key player in raising blood cholesterol and your risk of heart disease. Saturated fat is mainly found in meat, dairy products, and oils like coconut, palm, and palm kernel oils. Watch out for Trans Fats in baked goods. Trans Fats will not appear on the label. Instead, look for hydrogenated or partial hydrogenated in the ingredients list.

- **Cholesterol:** Cholesterol is second cousin to fat. Challenge yourself to eat less than 200 mg each day.

- **Sodium:** Sodium is otherwise known as "salt." Either way, it may add up to high blood pressure in some people. Keep your sodium intake to 2,000 mg or less each day.

- **Daily Value:** This is a KEY number. % Daily Value shows how a food fits into the overall diet of 2,000 calories a day. For the categories of fat, saturated fat, cholesterol, and sodium choose foods with a LOW % Daily Value. For the categories of total carbohydrates, dietary fiber, vitamins and minerals your goal is to reach 100%. (See RDA Chart that follows)

- **Sugars:** Keep simple sugars as low as possible. Remember 1 teaspoon equals 16 calories.

BASIC RULES:

1. Daily Values: Try to limit fat, particularly saturated and trans fat, cholesterol, and sodium. Try to reach a daily goal of 100% for total carbohydrate, dietary fiber, vitamins and minerals.

2. Label ingredients: The ingredients are listed by weight with the ingredient present in the largest quantity listed first, the next largest quantity next and so forth. Check out your labels to see if they have sugar, fat, or sodium listed in more than one way.

3. The confusing part about labels is they list protein, carbohydrate and fat nutrients in grams, rather than calories. To know how many calories of protein, carbohydrate, and fat you are eating, you must learn how to convert grams to calories.

GENERAL RULE: If the percentages are NOT listed, chances are it is NOT a healthy product!

LABELS DON'T LIE, BUT LIARS MAKE LABELS.

RDA — RECOMMENDED DAILY ALLOWANCE

- **TOTAL FAT**   <25%
- **SATURATED FAT**   <10%
- **CHOLESTEROL**   <200 mg
- **SODIUM**   <2,000 mg
- **DIETARY FIBER**   >38 g (men) >23 g (women)
- **SUGARS (SIMPLE)**   <15 %
- **PROTEIN**   <15%

For a chart of RDA's, go to www.nal.usda.gov/fnic/dga/rda.pdf

ENERGY CONVERSION

*To convert grams of protein and carbohydrate to calories, multiply the grams by 4.
To convert grams of fat to calories, multiply the grams by 9.*

READING THE NUTRITION LABEL

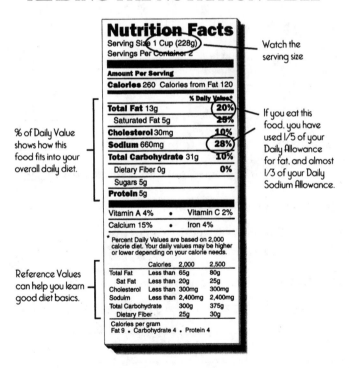

Contrary to what you may have been led to believe, this label does not tell you the precent of fat in this food. To learn this information, you must divide the calories per serving (260) into the calories from fat (120). This food is 46% fat!

LABEL READING WORKSHEET

REMEMBER: 1 gram of protein = 4 calories
1 gram of carbohydrates = 4 calories
1 gram of fat = 9 calories
1 gram of alcohol = 7 calories

LOWFAT COTTAGE CHEESE: *Nutrient Information per serving*

Serving size ....1/2 cup
Servings per container...........4
Calories................................100
Protein ....14 grams
Carbohydrates......................4 grams
Fat.......................................2 grams

INGREDIENTS: Grade A cultured nonfat milk, milk, milk cream, salt, annatto extract, acetic acid.

1. What size is each serving? _____

2. How many servings in the whole container? _____

3. How many calories in each serving? _____

4. How many calories in the whole container? _____

5. Of the calories, how many come from protein? (14x4)_____

6. Of the calories, how many come from carbohydrates? (4x4)_____

7. Of the calories, how many come from fat? (2x9)_____

8. What PERCENT of the 100 calories comes from fat? _____
    (divide fat calories by total calories per serving)

9. Is this a lowfat food? _____

10. Is there any reason to avoid this food in a balanced and varied, low fat, low sugar, high fiber diet? _____

    If so, what is it? _____

1: 1/2 cup 2: 4 serv. 3: 100 cal. 4: 400 cal. 5: 56 cal. 6: 16 cal. 7: 18 cal. 8: 18%

BUILD IT AND THEY WILL COME!
SEE IT AND YOU WILL BUY IT! BUY IT AND YOU WILL EAT IT!

A few years ago there was a movie "Field of Dreams" starring Kevin Costner. He heard a message that if he built a baseball field in his cornfield in Iowa, the old time baseball players, Ruth, Cobb, Speaker, etc. would come to play.

The other day I was in the supermarket where I made several spur of the moment purchases that I knew I would regret, seeing that once I buy something, I don't have the willpower to throw it away. My mother taught me at an early age to eat all the food on my plate as people around the world were starving to death.

Therefore, I have resolved to have a shopping list before I go into the store and follow it to the letter. To assist in making healthy selections I would suggest Evelyn Kissinger's "Healthy Shopping" video. See the Appendix for purchasing information.

RULE 9. WATCH YOUR SERVING SIZES

This is the major dietary problem in our society today. We are now in the age of the 64 oz. "Double Gulp," 32 oz. "Slurpee" soda drink or the 39¢ "Super Size" which adds 50% more fat and doubles the calories to your "Value Meal." Remember, "We can pay the price now (through using discipline and not 'supersizing' the meal) or pay the bigger price later with a heart attack."

Studies show that most overweight people tend to misjudge their daily caloric count by underestimating the serving size. Also, people seem more able to choose the appropriate portion size when they compare it to a nonfood object such as a deck of cards, a golf ball, or a domino. People were more accurate when they were linking serving size to a visual cue than to the actual portion. The American Dietetic Association has endorsed this idea of "visual cue" and published a guide to help end "portion distortion."

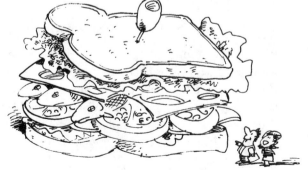

A SERVING IS A LOT LESS THAN YOU THINK!

STANDARD SERVINGS:

Golf Ball = 1 ounce of meatball

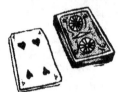

Deck of Cards = 3 ounces of cooked lean meat (1 serving)

Baseball = 1 cup of milk or yogurt

3 Dominos = 1 1/2 ounces of cheese

1 SERVING

Bread..................... 1 slice

Cereal..................... 1 cup

Vegetables............... 1/2 cup cooked, 1 cup raw.

Fruit..................... 1 medium piece, 4 oz. juice

Meat..................... 3-4 oz.

Nuts..................... 1 small handful

Dairy..................... 1 - 8 oz. glass of milk; 1 - 8 oz. Yogurt; 1-2 oz. cheese

NUTRITION TIPS: Divide your plate and make it colorful

Pretend your dinner plate is divided into four quarters. Fill three of the quarters with grains, vegetables, legumes (peas or beans), and/or fruits and only one quarter with meat. You'll get the correct mix of nutrients, control portion sizes, and cut fat and calories. The key is to have a variety of food and watch your portion sizes. "Too much on your plate" applies to more than a busy lifestyle. Even lean foods can sabotage your good intentions if your portions are oversized. Developing an eye for size is your best defense.

Another guideline is to make your plate as colorful as possible. See how many colors you can get on the plate (ketchup on your fries doesn't count). For example, try filling your plate with green for beans, orange for sweet potato, blue for blueberries and red for strawberries.

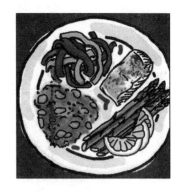

RULE 10. MAKE "GOOD" CHOICES WHEN EATING OUT

My first inclination as I wrote this dietary rule was to discourage eating out, especially at fast food restaurants, as most of the meals tend to be extremely high in fat, sodium and sugar. Plus, there's little control over the method of preparation (trans fats to prepare the french fries), little knowledge of the nutritional value of the food, and a tendency to make impulsive selections (high calorie dessert). To top it off, we "supersize" and add twice the fat and calories for less than fifty cents. The two most dangerous words in the English language are "Super Size!"

There used to be trucks carrying oil filters that had the following words written on the side of the trailer: "You can pay the price now (meaning oil changes) or pay later (new engine)." We will certainly pay the big "Super Size" price later in increased health costs and diminished quality of life, unless we resist this "Super Sizing" temptation. The biggest selling item in the restaurant supply business is the 12 & 14 inch plate, because the 10 inch plate won't hold the food anymore.

In the 1950's only 5% of our meals were eaten out and we had to search to find a fast food restaurant. Americans spent a scant 19 percent of their food dollar on food that was prepared outside the home. Today over 50% of our meals are eaten out, we spend 41 percent of our food dollar on outside food, and there is a fast food restaurant on every corner. The fast food industry is now a 222 billion dollar industry, with over 50% of that spent in the drive-thru lane. McDonald's is the leader at over 20 billion restaurants in more than 13,500 cities in the U.S.

NOT AN ANTI-AGING DIET. *Morgan Sprulock, a New York filmmaker, made a documentary in which he filmed himself during a month of eating every meal at McDonald's. At 6'2" and 185 lbs., Spurlock is a non smoker, non drinker, and exercises daily. During the making of the film, "Super Size Me," he gained 25 pounds, his cholesterol climbed from 165 to 230, his liver began to fail, his skin turned splotchy, and he lost his sex drive.*

How many people know that a typical taco salad harbors as much fat as 18 strips of bacon? A dinner of prime rib, Caesar salad and loaded baked potato is one of the least nutritious meals on the planet? The famous Bloomin' Onion with dipping sauce packs a whopping 2,130 calories. Unfortunately, when the FDA in 1994 required food you purchased in the supermarket to have nutrition breakdowns, they did not require labels on restaurant food.

A good guide to restaurants is the book, Restaurant Confidential. It gives a breakdown by restaurant category: Mexican, Italian, Chinese, seafood, pizzeria, steakhouse, etc. There is a "Restaurant Hall of Fame," listing healthy food choices and a "Restaurant Hall of Shame," which lists the not-so healthy choices. (Jacobson)

BEST RESTAURANT MEALS

- The Olive Garden - Chicken Giardino and minestrone soup
- Denny's Slim Slam - (Egg Beaters, ham, two hotcakes with fruit topping)
- Grilled chicken or seafood, baked potato with sour cream and vegetable
- Pasta with marinara or clam sauce and salad with light dressing
- Subway - "7 under 7" sub and baked potato chips
- Au Bon Plain bagel with preserves and yogurt with berries

Some of these same restaurants also made the "Hall of Shame" list. Olive Garden features a Fettuccine Alfredo at 1,500 calories that was dubbed "heart attack on a plate." The same Olive Garden menu features the Chicken Giardino mentioned above. As always, it comes down to CHOICES, which is what this book is all about.

Fast food restaurants are even popping up in schools and hospitals. In St. Louis, Missouri, there is a school system of 27,000 students where the students can bring a sack lunch or on Mondays have McDonald's, Tuesday's Domino's Pizza, Wednesday Taco Bell, Thursday Subway, and Friday Pizza Hut. The breakfast special Monday thru Friday 7-10 am is Dunkin' Donuts. Is it any wonder that our children are the heaviest in the world?

SCHOOL LUNCHES

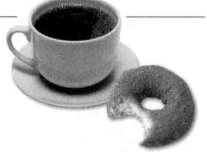

Monday ....McDonald's
Tuesday ....Domino's Pizza
Wednesday ....Taco Bell
Thursday........................Subway
Friday............................Pizza Hut

BREAKFAST SPECIAL (Mon-Fri, 7-10 am): Coffee and Dunkin' Donuts!

154

The fast food industry has even invaded what should be the most health conscious places in the country – the hospitals. In a recent survey, six of the nation's 16 top hospitals had onsite fast food restaurants. One of the researchers said that the high calorie havens send mixed messages to hospital patients, visitors, and employees. On one hand, we say obesity is linked to fast food and at the same time we make it easy to get in health institutions.

If we can't escape the fast food scene, then the next option is to make "intelligent choices." If you look closely at most restaurants, you can usually find some healthy options. My favorite fast food restaurant is Subway. I've found that their 6" "Veggie Delite" on wheat is only 230 calories with only 3 grams of fat.. Compare that to a Big Mac at McDonald's at 590 calories and 34 grams of fat. Even the 6" turkey breast is only 280 calories and 4.5 grams of fat. Subway has eight subs under 311 calories.

Healthy Fast Food Options

	Calories	Fat (gms)
SUBWAY (8 Varieties – 6" subs)	200-311	2.5 - 4.5
PIZZA HUT (Veggie – 1 slice)	22	8
MCDONALD'S (Grilled Chicken)	300	5
WENDY'S (Chili – large)	310	10

Above information from Nutrition in the Fast Lane, This inexpensive, pocket sized book is updated every year. For ordering information, call Rainbow Wellness: 269-925-3524.

RULE 11. SELECT "TRAFFIC LIGHT" FOODS

The other day I was doing a crossword puzzle, and they wanted a four letter word for "food fad." The answer was diet. Unfortunately, that is what most people view diets as, a fad that they do for a short period and discard when something else comes along. A diet should be viewed as a life-long eating plan. That is why I've shied away from including diets in my books. All of us have different food preferences.

People ask to have a food plan laid out for them. With over 30,000 food items and everyone coming from different backgrounds and ethnic origins, whatever diet I prescribe for you will probably not be something you can follow. That is why I like Oldway's "EatWise" Pyramid. It allows you to make your own selections, based upon your desires.

I recently came across the "Stoplight Eating Plan" which makes a lot of sense. It has been developed by the University of Pittsburgh and funded by the National Institutes of Health and has more than a 10-year track record with impressive successes. At least one third of the participants have maintained a healthy body weight 10 years after beginning the program.

Concept: Food is divided into three groups patterned after the colors on a traffic light – red, yellow and green. Studies show that people who feel deprived of their favorite food don't succeed at weight loss, however there are no forbidden foods on this diet. Foods high in fat and calories are "red" foods which should be eaten very sparingly. While "yellow" foods are more healthy than "red" foods, they too shouldn't be eaten in large quantities. They are moderate-calorie, moderate-fat foods and are given the color "yellow." You get a "green" light for LOW-FAT, LOW CALORIE foods. As with any eating plan, portion control is paramount. Again, avoiding the "red" foods doesn't mean that you never have them, just sparingly, such as once or twice a week. There is no such thing as "forbidden" food.

TRAFFIC LIGHT FOODS

List below your "red," "yellow" and "green" foods. These foods will change as your taste preferences change.

RED – STOP!

_____   _____
_____   _____
_____   _____

YELLOW – CAUTION

_____   _____
_____   _____
_____   _____

GREEN – GO

_____   _____
_____   _____
_____   _____

RULE 12. CONSIDER SUPPLEMENTATION

More than three-quarters of Americans take some form of dietary supplement to maintain good health and enhance inadequate diets. The supplement industry has become a multi-billion dollar industry. Individuals need to be knowledgeable about various treatment options, and, with their doctor's help, choose those options that are best suited for them. In the next chapter, some of these options will be discussed.

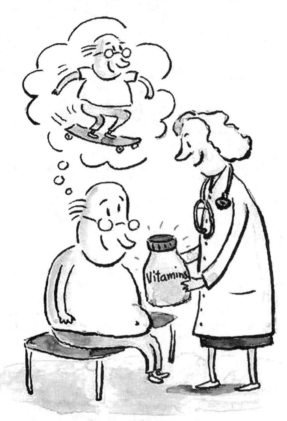

SLIMMING SOFTWARE

Can't afford a full time nutritionist and physical trainer? The award-winning DINE program ($129 plus s&h) was introduced in 1982 and, twenty-two years later, it is still the leader. You can design your own eating and exercise program. The database includes more than 10,000 foods enabling you to design a 7-day sample meal plan, along with an analysis of your physical activity level. The best feature of the program is the DINE score, an index that tells you how well (or how poorly) you're eating. (800-688-1848 or www.dinesystems.com)

WHAT IS YOUR
NUTRITIONAL SCOREBOARD?

FOOD GROUP	Monday	Tuesday	Wednesday
WHOLE GRAINS: _____ servings. *1 slice bread; 1/2 bun; 1 bagel or English muffin; 1 oz. dry, ready-to-eat cereal; 1/2 cup cooked cereal, rice or pasta.*	Goal:_____ Actual:_____	Goal:_____ Actual:_____	Goal:_____ Actual:_____
VEGETABLES: _____ servings. *1 cup raw leafy greens; 1/2 cup other kinds of vegetables.*	Goal:_____ Actual:_____	Goal:_____ Actual:_____	Goal:_____ Actual:_____
FRUIT: _____ servings. *1 medium apple, orange or banana; 3/4 cup juice; 1/2 cup small or diced fruit; 1/4 cup dried fruit.*	Goal:_____ Actual:_____	Goal:_____ Actual:_____	Goal:_____ Actual:_____
LOW FAT/SKIM MILK: _____ servings. *1 cup milk or yogurt; 1 1/2 oz. cheese; 1 cup ice cream, ice milk or frozen yogurt.*	Goal:_____ Actual:_____	Goal:_____ Actual:_____	Goal:_____ Actual:_____
MEAT OR MEAT SUBSTITUTES: No more than 6 oz. *3 oz. cooked lean meat, poultry or fish; The following items equal 1 oz. of mean: 1/2 cup cooked beans; 1 egg; 2 Tbs. peanut butter; 4 oz. tofu (2 oz. extra firm); 1/4 cup nuts or seeds.*	Goal:_____ Actual:_____	Goal:_____ Actual:_____	Goal:_____ Actual:_____
FAT – 1 TABLESPOON: *Oil, butter, margarine, salad dressing, mayonnaise., corn oil, olive oil.*	Goal:_____ Actual:_____	Goal:_____ Actual:_____	Goal:_____ Actual:_____
SWEETS – NO MORE THAN 1 PER DAY	Goal:_____ Actual:_____	Goal:_____ Actual:_____	Goal:_____ Actual:_____

Thursday	Friday	Saturday	Sunday	Weekly Totals
Goal:_____ Actual:_____	Goal:_____ Actual:_____	Goal:_____ Actual:_____	Goal:_____ Actual:_____	Goal:_____ Actual:_____
Goal:_____ Actual:_____	Goal:_____ Actual:_____	Goal:_____ Actual:_____	Goal:_____ Actual:_____	Goal:_____ Actual:_____
Goal:_____ Actual:_____	Goal:_____ Actual:_____	Goal:_____ Actual:_____	Goal:_____ Actual:_____	Goal:_____ Actual:_____
Goal:_____ Actual:_____	Goal:_____ Actual:_____	Goal:_____ Actual:_____	Goal:_____ Actual:_____	Goal:_____ Actual:_____
Goal:_____ Actual:_____	Goal:_____ Actual:_____	Goal:_____ Actual:_____	Goal:_____ Actual:_____	Goal: < 42 oz. Actual:_____
Goal:_____ Actual:_____	Goal:_____ Actual:_____	Goal:_____ Actual:_____	Goal:_____ Actual:_____	Goal: ≤ 7Tbs. Actual:_____
Goal:_____ Actual:_____	Goal:_____ Actual:_____	Goal:_____ Actual:_____	Goal:_____ Actual:_____	Goal: ≤ 7 Actual:_____

RATE YOUR PLATE

Using the "EatWise" Pyramid in chapter 7 and the 12 Dietary Rules in the beginning of this chapter, list a daily food plan that you can eat for the rest of your life.

BREAKFAST			
ENTRÉE	SERVING SIZE	CALORIES	FAT (GRAMS)
Comments:			
LUNCH			
Comments:			
DINNER			
Comments:			
SNACKS			
Comments:			
		TOTAL CAL.	TOTAL FAT
Breakfast			
Lunch			
Dinner			
Snacks			
TOTALS			

TOTAL FAT CALORIES: _____ (Fat grams X 9 calories)

% of Fat: _____ (Fat calories /Total calories)

NOTE: Don't use one day as a representative of daily food intake. Take 3 different days and average them to get an accurate picture. What grade (A, B, C, D, or E) would you give this plate? What changes can you make to improve the grade?

CHAPTER NINE

SUPPLEMENTATION

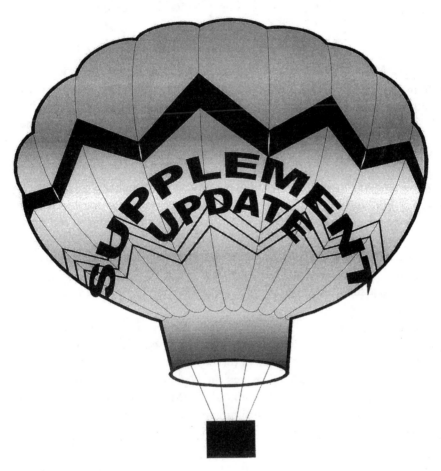

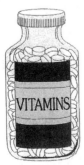

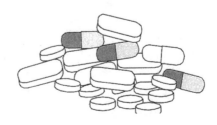

SUPPLEMENTATION

"My advice concerns diet ... along with intelligent use of vitamins, supplements and herbs. You can really help your body by taking protective anti-oxidants, nutrients that protect tissues." — Andrew Weil, MD, author

> SUPPLEMENTATION: According to the Dietary Supplement Health and Education Act (DSHEA), 1994, a supplement is a dietary product taken by mouth that contains dietary ingredient(s) intended to supplement the diet. Such ingredients include vitamins, minerals, herbs, or other botanicals, amino acids, and substances such as enzymes, organ tissues, glandulars, and metabolites.

Supplementation has become an industry in excess of 19 billion dollars, with more than 1,000 companies producing products ranging from mainstream vitamins to herbs, to controversial hormones and stimulants. While most companies are credible, unfortunately there are some unscrupulous companies, again "buyer-beware." By most estimates, a vast majority of Americans are using nutritional supplements. It is estimated that over 60 million Americans are taking nutritional supplements. According to a 2001 AARP survey, 52% of people 50 and older take a supplement.

Everyone recognizes that alternative therapies are widely used and are of value. However, many are unproven, and many change a body function so they MUST be thought of in the same way as any other medication. To address these issues, the National Institutes of Health has created the National Center for Complementary and Alternative Medicine (NCCAM). NCCAM currently has several studies underway, and, hopefully, in the near future we will have much more information on alternative therapies. They are looking at the entire field of alternative medicine.

The problem is that there is a voluminous amount of information out there, and it is hard to separate fact from fiction. Knowledge is power – power to control decisions that influence your wellness and mold your future. Nowhere in wellness is knowledge more important than in the selection of vitamins, minerals, and herbs. Your choices can literally mean the difference between life and death. Be sure your knowledge is coming from reputable sources.

The fact is that each of us are biologically unique. We all share the same basic cellular structure, but our individual combination of genes makes us unlike anyone else who has lived. As Dr. George Sheehan, the cardiologist and marathon runner used to say, "We are all an experiment of one." We all have our own biological needs and our own responses to the world around us. What works for one person may not work for another.

It is impossible in the limited scope of this book to adequately cover this broad topic. My hope is that, by reading the basic information I've provided, you will spend time researching this important topic. The use of any nutritional supplement should not be undertaken without the approval of a knowledgeable health professional. There are many dangers in self diagnosing. If you are currently taking prescription medicine, you MUST work with your physician before altering any drug regimen. Unfortunately, because vitamins and minerals are classified under foods rather than drugs, they are not subjected to the intense scrutiny and testing that drugs receive. For this reason, it is essential that you fully check out all supplements before using them. It is a mistake to assume that because something is natural, it is also safe! For further information on this field of natural nutrition, I would suggest the following resources:

- **National Institute of Health, Center for Complementary and Alternative Medicine (NCCAM)** 888-644-6226. www.nccam.nih.gov. Call and request a general packet of information on complementary and alternative medicine. (CAM)

- **Prescription for Nutritional Healing**, 3rd edition. Phyllis A. Balch, CNC and James F Balch, MD, (Avery Publishing) ISBN: 1-58333-077-1, 2000. (Many consider this to be the "Bible" of supplements).

- **The ABC Clinical Guide to Herbs**, (American Botanical Council). This book covers uses, dosages, adverse effects and drug interactions. To order, call 1-800-373-7105.

- **ConsumerLab.com**. An independent company that tests herbal, vitamin, and mineral supplements. Found at: www.consumerlab.com

One of the major problems with vitamins, herbs, and other nutritional supplements is the poor product quality. Neither the U.S. government nor any other government agency is responsible for testing dietary supplements for their contents or quality. Products can remain on store shelves for months or even years before they are sold. In addition to selecting a product that looks like it has the right ingredients, there is no guarantee that it contains what it claims, that it breaks down properly once in the body, or that it is free of impurities.

ConsumerLab.com is an independent and quality testing company based in White Plains, NY, which tests supplements to see if they contain the quantity of active ingredients listed on their label. In 2001, they tested 27 multi-vitamin products. Nine failed to contain the amounts listed, and four had amounts that exceeded the recommended levels of upper intake. Thus, half of the products tested did not meet accepted standards.

ConsumerLab.com is constantly testing different supplements, and their results can be viewed on their subscription based web site. The cost for a year's subscription is quite minimal, especially when it concerns your body!

In March 2003, the U.S. Food and Drug Administration (FDA) took steps to help consumers get uncontaminated and better-labeled products. Hopefully, these changes will require the manufacturers to list the amount and strength of their ingredients. In the meantime, this continues to be a buyers-beware market.

HOW TO CHOOSE A SUPPLEMENT

- Look for nationally known food and supplement companies.
- Look for products that have recognized symbols of quality such as USP or ConsumerLabs.com.
- Avoid foreign products unless quality is known.
- Avoid companies that make sensational claims or have misleading or vague labeling.
- Look for products that have standardized extracts.
- Look for products that have an expiration date.
- Look for products that provide a toll-free customer service phone number.
- Check to see if they have any published studies supporting their use.

SUPPLEMENTS

Like water, carbohydrates, proteins, fats, vitamins, and minerals are essential to life. The U.S. Food and Drug Administration (FDA) has formulated consumption levels called recommended daily allowances (RDA). However, these levels were formulated almost 50 years ago, and they do not account for the amount needed to maintain maximum health. They are the minimums necessary to prevent deficiency diseases such as rickets, beriberi, scurvy, and night blindness.

For further reading on the recommendations, see, Dietary Reference Intakes for Vitamin C, Vitamin E, Selenium and Carotenoids, (Institute of Medicine, Washington Academy Press, Washington, D.C., 2000).

According to James F. Balch, MD, author of Prescription for Nutritional Healing, "People who are active and exercise, those who are under great stress, on restricted diets, mentally or physically ill, women who take oral contraceptives, those on medication, those who are recovering from surgery, smokers and those who consume alcoholic beverages all need higher than normal amounts of nutrients." (Balch)

As I alluded to in the beginning, ideally, there should be no need for supplementation. We know what foods we should eat, we know that exercise is essential to a healthy body, and finally we know what stress does to our bodies. Despite knowing the importance of nutrition, exercise, and a positive attitude, it doesn't translate into doing it. Unfortunately, only 12% of Americans eat a healthy diet.

Due to our stressful way of life, supplementation is almost a necessity if we want to improve or even maintain our present levels of health. Because of the high consumption of fast foods, sugar, alcohol, tobacco and caffeine; the fact that we have taken movement out of our lives; and the fast paced lifestyles we lead, almost everyone has a need for supplementation. While most of us would like to eat a balanced diet, for a multitude of reasons we fall short of the goal. Neil Stone, MD (Chairman of the American Heart Assoc. Nutrition Committee) says, "Perhaps 5 of the 10 leading causes of death in the U.S. are nutritionally caused, and, as such, diseases like heart disease, cancer, and stroke can often be prevented."

Dr. Jeffrey Blumberg, Ph.D., Chief of Antioxidant Research Lab, Tufts University, encourages proper eating habits, but insists that supplementing with vitamins and minerals should be considered a low-cost form of health insurance. He says, "Wearing a seat belt doesn't give you a license to drive recklessly, it just protects you in case of an accident. Supplements work the same way. They don't give you a license to eat poorly and otherwise abuse your health, but they provide an added cushion of protection!"

Dr. Hans Diehl, developer of the worldwide Coronary Health Improvement Project (CHIP), author, and one of the leading alternative health experts in the country, makes a strong case for getting our vitamins the natural way – through our foods. He points out that if you daily eat a variety of fresh fruits, whole grains, and vegetables, your need for vitamins, minerals, and fiber is easily met. (Diehl)

VITAMINS

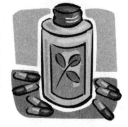

Vitamin A: A fat soluble vitamin that promotes healthy eyes, hair and skin, bone and tooth growth, is an antioxidant for cancer and heart disease.

Vitamin B Complex: **B1:** (thiamine) Enhances blood circulation, carbohydrate metabolism, improved brain function, internal muscle tone and acts as an antioxidant protecting the body against effects of aging, alcohol, and smoking.

B2: (riboflavin) Necessary for red blood cell formation, antibody production, cell respiration and growth, treatment of cataracts, skin, nails, and hair formation, important during pregnancy, and aids in the metabolism of fats, carbohydrates, and proteins.

B3: (niacin, niacinamide, and nicotinic acid) Necessary for proper circulation, metabolism of nutrients, lowering cholesterol, and production of bile and stomach fluids.

B5: (pantothenic acid) Known as the "anti-stress vitamin," aids in formation of antibodies, vitamin utilization, and conversion of nutrients into energy.

B6: (pyridoxine) Involved in more bodily functions than any other single nutrient. It affects physical and mental health, metabolism of nutrients, brain function, synthesis of RNA and DNA, activates many enzymes, plays a role in cancer immunity, inhibits the formation of a toxic chemical called homocysteine which attacks the heart muscle.

B12: (cyanocobalamin) Needed to prevent anemia, digestion of nutrition, cell formation, prevents nerve damage, and assists memory and learning.

Vitamin C: (ascorbic acid) Powerful antioxidant that is necessary for bone, muscle, and blood vessel growth, enhances immunity, promotes the healing of wounds and burns, and protects against the harmful effects of pollution.

Vitamin D: A fat soluble vitamin that is necessary for bone and teeth formation, maintenance of heart action and nervous system, enhances immunity, necessary for thyroid function and normal blood clotting.

Vitamin E: A fat soluble antioxidant that protects blood cells and body tissue from cancer and cardiovascular disease, improves circulation, necessary for tissue repair and many more functions.

Vitamin K: A fat soluble vitamin necessary for blood clotting, bone formation and repair, proper liver function.

Folic Acid: Folic acid is water soluble and works in partnership with Vitamin B12 in the development of the nervous system, cell division, and red blood cell formation. Considered a "brain food," impaired mental acuity (dementia) and depression are common symptoms of folic acid or B12 deficiency. Folic acid is also very important in pregnancy as it helps in the fetal nerve cell formation. Because it must be taken BEFORE pregnancy, it is recommended that every woman of child bearing age take a folic acid supplement daily as a matter of course.

Coenzyme Q10: While Q10 is not a vitamin, it does resemble Vitamin E, and it plays a critical role in the production of energy in every cell of the body. It aids the circulation, and immune systems, increases tissue oxygenation and has anti-aging properties. It has also been proven to be very effective in the treatment and prevention of cardiovascular disease. Many studies have shown that it strengthens the heart muscle, reduces high blood pressure, and enhances the immune system. The amount of Q10 in the body declines with age, so people over the age of 50 should consider supplementing their diet with Q10.

WARNING: One area that we must look out for are the differences between fat soluble and water soluble vitamins. Fat or oil soluble vitamins, such as A, D, E, and K, are soluble only in fat. Overloads cannot be excreted, but are picked up and stored in the body's fatty tissue and the liver. Over long periods of time, these excesses can become toxic. The water soluble vitamins (C and B) cannot be stored but must be taken into the body daily as they are excreted within 1-4 days.

VITAMIN C: GOOD OR BAD FOR YOUR HEART?

Vitamin C is the most widely used supplement. Study after study has shown the beneficial effects of this vitamin. In 1999 there was a small study that tended to disprove the benefits of this supplement. However, the medical experts feel that this was not a valid study and cite the following heart benefits from taking Vitamin C.

Reduces Artery Thickening: There are many studies that show this benefit. One of the biggest was a 1995 study involving 10,000 subjects in which it was found that those who got the most Vitamin C had the least thickening of carotid-artery walls.

Lowers Blood Pressure: Taking 500 mg Vitamin C daily cuts high blood pressure about 9% in a 1999 study which makes it as effective as common blood pressure drugs.

Improves Blood Flow: Recent studies have shown that taking 500 mg of Vitamin C helps normalize artery function, thus reducing odds of blood clot formation, plaque buildup, heart attack, and stroke.

Wipes Out the Artery-Clogging Effects of Homocysteine: At least three major studies in 1999 showed that taking 1000-2000 mg a day helped block the dangerous artery-destroying effects of homocysteine. Keeping homocysteine in check is considered critical in warding off cardiovascular disease.

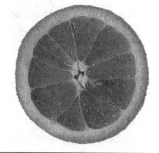

MINERALS

Minerals come from the earth, and it is important to obtain these essential elements. However, our food may be lacking in minerals because of the loss of top soil, continual replanting without enriching the soil, and by the farmers' use of fertilizers that contain only nitrogen, phosphorus, and potassium. Mineral deficiency is more common than vitamin deficiency because our bodies do not manufacture minerals and foods may be enriched with only vitamins and not minerals.

There are approximately 18 essential minerals – five are macro minerals, with the remainder being micro minerals or trace. The difference is that macro minerals are needed in larger amounts.

MACRO

Calcium: Necessary for healthy bone and muscle function.

Magnesium: Catalyst for enzymes involved in energy production.

Phosphorus: Necessary for bone and tooth formation, cell growth and contraction of heart muscle and kidney function.

Potassium: Helps maintain normal fluid balance and blood pressure.

Sodium: Assists in maintenance of proper water balance and blood ph.

As with vitamins, the healthy approach is to get the majority of minerals from foods. It is also necessary to assess your body's mineral content, state of health and lifestyle; then, after consultation with your knowledgeable physician, supplement accordingly.

FREE RADICALS AND ANTI-OXIDANTS

One of life's ironies is that the same oxygen that is essential for life can also cause serious damage to cells. Normal metabolism (breathing) and environmental contaminants (smoking, alcohol, pollutants, radiation) produce oxygen molecules in a highly reactive, unstable form known as "free radicals."

Excess free radicals may cause a chemical chain reaction producing more free radicals that can injure cells and genes by the process of oxidation. Each free radical may exist for only a fraction of a second, but the damage it leaves behind can be irreversible. This cell-destroying process contributes to as many as 51 different diseases from cataracts to cancer to hardening of the arteries. Free radicals are not all bad. We need them for essential functions such as destroying harmful viruses and bacteria, producing vital hormones needed for life, and producing energy. However, when the body starts producing free radicals in excess, damage to cells can occur.

Many factors can cause this excess production of free radicals.

- Exposure to radiation from sun or excessive medical x-rays.
- Environmental pollutants — tobacco smoke, car exhaust, unclean air.
- Diets high in fat. (This increases free radical activities, as oxidation occurs more readily in fat molecules than in carbohydrates and protein molecules.)
- Fried foods. (Frying in oil can produce large amounts of free radicals.)

This damaging process can be stopped or slowed down by antioxidants, which are vitamins, minerals, and other bio-chemicals made or taken in by our bodies that neutralize the harmful effects of the free radicals. Some examples of antioxidants are alpha-lipoic acid, bilberry, coenzyme Q10, homocysteine, ginkgo biloba, glutathine, grape seed extract, green tea, melatonin, selenium, Vitamin A and beta carotene, Vitamin C, Vitamin E, and zinc.

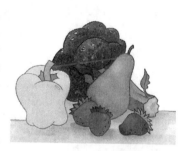

MEDICINAL (and delicious) FRUIT: POWERFUL BERRIES

Blueberries, cherries, grapes, and cranberries are emerging as the disease-fighting foods of the new millennium. In the past several years, researchers have discovered that drinking two glasses of Concord grape juice daily may be as beneficial as 400 IU of Vitamin E.

Blueberries

In a study by the USDA Human Nutrition Research Center on Aging at Tufts University, they discovered that blueberries ranked among the highest in antioxidants out of 40 vegetables, fruits and juices tested. Just a 1/2 cup of blueberries contained as many antioxidants as five servings of peas, carrots, apples, squash, and broccoli.

Luscious, sweet blueberries contain anthocyanin, the pigment that makes a blueberry blue and gives it the antioxidant power. Studies, conducted at Tufts University, Rutgers University, and the University of California at Davis, have shown that blueberries can prevent free radical damage to cells in the body. They can reverse short term memory loss and other effects of aging Blueberries can reduce urinary tract infections and LDL (bad) cholesterol In addition, a one cup serving will give you 5 grams of fiber and 15% of your daily Vitamin C requirement - all at only 80 calories. PRETTY IMPRESSIVE FOR A SMALL BERRY!!

Grapes

Researchers at the University of Texas found that two glasses of Concord grape juice had qualities similar to Vitamin E. The most notable feature was the ability of the grape juice flavonoids to oxidize the LDL (bad) cholesterol (10% reduction). In addition, grape juice produced a 20% decrease in the oxidation of plasma proteins, a benefit that was not exhibited by Vitamin E.

WE CAN NOW GET THE HEALTH BENEFIT ATTRIBUTED TO WINE WITHOUT THE ALCOHOL

Cherries

Drinking an 8 ounce glass of cherry juice on a daily basis helps control arthritis, gout, joint pain, lower LDL cholesterol, strengthen the immune system, inhibit the growth of colon cancer tumors, and many more benefits. I can personally attest to the arthritis health benefit as I've been using it for several years with good results.

Researchers at Michigan State University, University of Texas, University of Iowa, Brunswick Laboratories, and the Medical University of South Carolina have demonstrated that the pigment called anthocyanin is truly "Mother Nature's all natural chemotherapy agent." In addition to anthocyanin, cherries have two flavonoids, isoqueritrin and queritrin, that are some of the most potent anticancer agents ever discovered.

In addition to Montmorency tart cherries being nutritious and great tasting, they're naturally high in potassium, low in fat, calories, and sodium. In addition, cherries are high in natural melatonin, which is well known to improve sleep patterns.

All you have to do is add two tablespoons (one ounce) of Montmorency concentrate to a glass of water, cola, spritzer, etc., and you'll get the power of 60 fresh tart cherries.

CHERRY YOGURT SMOOTHIE

1 cup non-fat plain or vanilla yogurt
1 ripe banana, peeled and sliced
1/2 cup orange juice
2-4 tablespoons of tart cherry juice concentrate
1 cup crushed ice

Put above mixture in electric blender and puree until smooth. Makes two 8 oz servings.

Cranberries

Besides being a good source of Vitamin C, cranberries have long been a favorite for treating mild urinary tract infections. Cranberries work by helping to prevent bacteria from adhering to the bladder's lining. Since sugar can exacerbate urinary tract infections, it's important to take the fruit in capsule form or as unsweetened juice if you have an active infection. As to the heart benefit, you have to drink an 8 ounce glass of low-sugar cranberry juice three times a day.

NOTE: Cranberries, blueberries, raspberries, bilberries, and blackberries come from similar families so it would seem logical to try and include all of them in our diet whenever possible. Raspberries are rich in niacin and potassium and have shown that they help inhibit the growth of cancer cells. Bilberries have been used in Europe for centuries for the improvement of vision and the prevention of cataracts. Blackberries have antioxidant qualities similar to blueberries.

MOST POWERFUL PRODUCE

When you're shopping for fruits and vegetables, keep in mind that phytochemicals in the pigments of deeply colored varieties can help protect against cancer and other diseases. The fruits and vegetables with the highest antioxidant potential (Oxygen Radical Absorbance Capacity or ORAC) are listed below.

Antioxidants

Fruits (raw)	Amount	ORAC
Prunes	4	1,939
Blueberries	1/2 cup	1,740
Blackberries	1/2 cup	1,466
Strawberries	1/2 cup	1,170
Raisins	1/4 cup	1,026
Raspberries	1/2 cup	756
Oranges	1/2 cup	675
Plums	1	626
Red Grapes	1/2 cup	591

Vegetables (raw)	Amount	ORAC
Kale	1 cup	1,186
Beets	1/2 cup	571
Red Bell Peppers	1/2 cup	533
Brussels Sprouts	1/2 cup	431
Yellow Corn	1/2 cup	420
Spinach	1 cup	378
Onions	1/2 cup	360
Broccoli Florets	1/2 cup	320
Eggplant	1 cup	320

USDA Agricultural Research Service.

HERBAL SUPPLEMENTS

Herbs have long been used for medicinal and nutritional purposes. Nutritionally, they have been used as food enhancers, extracts, vinegars, syrups, and in teas. Medicinally, they have been used for centuries in compresses, poultices, salves, and tinctures. There are over 100 commonly used medicinal herbs, and it is in this use that many medical authorities have concern. Unfortunately, herbal supplements are marketed for performance enhancement, weight loss, better health, and a growing list of other purposes. In many of these areas, there is no proof of their effectiveness.

As is the case with vitamins, herbal supplements are considered dietary supplements; thus they reach the market without meeting the safety and efficacy standards that the Food and Drug Administration (FDA) requires of over-the-counter and prescription medicine. Their potency and purity can vary from what is noted on the label. This means that for most herbs, the safe upper limit of dosage has not been determined, nor have their side effects, toxicity, long-term safety, and efficacy been determined. Thus, buyer beware (caveat emptor)!

In general, herbal medicines are far gentler than prescribed drugs. They work by supporting and strengthening the tissues and systems of the body rather than by radically changing them. In many situations, the appropriate dosage will be a blend of 3-6 different herbs. Therefore, it is essential to consult a medical herbalist who has been trained in orthodox diagnosis, as well as in the herbal pharmacopoeia. He/she will take into account a person's age, diet, lifestyle, and drug and medical history when deciding how best to support the body's restoration of health. Often this means identifying the underlying cause of ill health, rather than simply treating the symptoms. One reputable source on herbal products is www.herbalgram.org.

Many people think that a dietary supplement such as an herb is a food and has nothing to do with a drug. For example, is garlic a food or an herbal drug? The correct answer is that it's both. Some herbs have potent active components that act like prescription drugs. Because of this, herbs must be used appropriately, not indiscriminately. Doctors need to know what supplements their patients take because of their effects on the ability to clot blood or maintain blood pressure as well as interactions with prescribed medicine. For example, Echinacea, which is commonly used to fight colds, and St. John's Wort, an herb with mild sedative effects, pose a risk of bleeding and cardiovascular instability during surgery.

Herbs and surgery sometimes don't mix

Americans spend over four billion a year on herbal medicine. While the medical establishment is still largely skeptical about herbs citing a lack of scientific data, allergic reactions, side effects, and potentially dangerous interactions with other medicines, doctors as a rule are becoming more supportive.

A study by the University of Chicago shows that some common herbs can cause post surgical complications, and it is imperative that you inform your surgeon BEFORE you go to the hospital. Many supplements, not only herbs, but other common medications such as blood thinning agents like aspirin, Plavix, etc. require their stoppage 7-10 days before surgery. The researchers focused on the six most commonly used herbs in the U.S.

Herb	Possible Post-Surgery Effects	When to Stop
Ephedra	Increased blood pressure and heart rate	24 hours before surgery
Garlic	Inhibited blood clotting	1 week before surgery
Ginkgo	Inhibited blood clotting	24 hours before surgery
Kava	Can amplify the effects of anesthesia	24 hours before surgery
St. Johns Wort	Could interfere with post-op drugs	1 week before surgery
Valerian	Can amplify the effects of anesthesia	24 hours before surgery

NOTE: This list is not all-inclusive and is not intended to discourage you from taking herbs but rather to err on the side of caution in making sure that they're safe.

A recent survey of 46,000 Consumer Reports readers who use alternative therapies found that only 60% told their doctors that they used them. This can be dangerous! (Consumers Report).

BOTTOM LINE: You should always inform your doctor about ALL drugs you're taking – prescribed and over-the-counter. My wife and I have put all of our medications and surgeries into a spreadsheet which we can hand the nurse or emergency medical technician.

READ MORE ABOUT HERBS:

The Green Pharmacy, James Duke (Rodale Press, 1997)
The Herbal Drugstore, Linda White (Rodale Press, 2000)
The Encyclopedia of Popular Herbs, Robert McCaleb (Prima Pub, 2000)
The New Healing Herbs, Michael Castleman (Rodale Press, 2001)

NATURAL SUPPLEMENTS

Caution is also indicated for natural food supplements such as acidophilus, alfalfa, fish oil, flaxseed oil, grape seed oil, brans (oat, wheat, rice, psyllium and pectin), glucosamine, honey, melatonin, wheat germ, and many more. Many food supplements like aloe vera, garlic, saw palmetto, ginseng, primrose oil, and ginkgo biloba are listed as both an herb and a food supplement.

Acidophilus is known as a "friendly" bacteria that aids in digestion and the absorption of nutrients. Aloe Vera is well known for its healing effect and is used in many cosmetic and hair products. Fish oil is a good source of omega-3 fatty acids which are needed for proper body function. Ginkgo Biloba is known as the "brain" food. Studies show that it may boost memory and increase the supply of oxygen to the heart, brain and other body parts. Ginseng has been used in the Far East for centuries to combat weakness and fatigue and give extra energy.

There are two supplements that I can personally attest to. However, remember as I mentioned earlier, I am only an experiment of one and what has worked for me may not work for you. Again, as I've emphasized so many times in this chapter, check with a reputable health professional before you try any food or vitamin supplement.

My experience with these supplements is what scientists call anecdotal. It is a report of one person's experiences when he/she tried a certain treatment or therapy. The anecdote tells what the person perceived was happening which may or may not be what actually happened. Scientists don't rely on anecdotal evidence but on large randomized, double blind, clinical studies. The problem with supplements is that because they are so inexpensive, it does not pay a drug company to spend millions of dollars on a large study.

The first supplement I can recommend is glucosamine to relieve the pain of osteoarthritis. Glucosamine acts to protect and promote the growth of joint cartilage. As I mentioned in the beginning of the book, I've had both hips replaced, in fact I have considerable arthritis in my body. I was faced with taking non-steroidal, anti-inflammatory drugs (NSAID) for the rest of my life. This was not a pleasant thought as NSAID's have a lot of undesirable side effects. However, I've been taking 1500 mg of glucosamine and 1200 mg of chondroitin sulfate for the past eight years in place of the NSAID. While glucosamine is an amino sugar with no toxic or side effects, the same can not be said for chondroitin as it is chemically similar to heparin (blood thinner), and it can interact with other medications like aspirin.

If you have concerns about using chondroitin sulfate, you may want to consider the herb boswella and glucosamine. Studies are showing that this combination is effective without side effects.

There have been over 300 double blind studies and 20 clinical trials that show the effectiveness of this regimen. The Arthritis Foundation has declared this treatment as effective as the conventional NSAID's, such as ibuprofen, Advil, Motrin, Orudis, Feldene, and the others. Studies show that this combination reduces inflammation and even repairs cartilage. If it is going to help, you should see an improvement after two months. It has been my experience in talking to fellow arthritis sufferers that for many, glucosamine is a miracle drug. Since it is relatively inexpensive, with no known side effects, if it doesn't work all you're out is a few bucks. (Arthritis Foundation)

Another effective supplement for me is saw palmetto which has been widely used in Europe for the treatment of enlarged prostate, commonly referred to as "benign prostate hyperplasia" (BPH). Many studies have shown that it inhibits the production of a hormone that contributes to the enlargement of the prostate. Studies show a success rate of up to 90% and, unlike pharmaceutical drugs, virtually no side effects.

At the risk of getting egg on my face, I'm going to look into my crystal ball and list what at the time of writing this book appears to be the most effective natural supplements. Because this is a constantly changing field, tomorrow could completely change things – but I don't think so, as these supplements have undergone considerable scrutiny.

DON'S "NON-SCIENTIFIC" LIST OF THE TOP SUPPLEMENTS (In alphabetical order)

This list is unscientific but clearly shows the multitude of supplements available. I surveyed many books on natural medicine and supplements and took the most frequently mentioned, several of which I've personally experienced.

Aloe Vera: Applied externally to relieve painful sunburns, skin cuts, and various skin diseases.

Berries: Function as antioxidants, sleep aids, infection and glaucoma fighters (bilberries, blueberries, cherries, cranberries, grapes, hawthorn, strawberries, etc).

Coenzyme Q10: Prevents heart disease, diabetes, and high blood pressure.

Echinacea: Taken at onset of cold symptoms, cuts both the severity and length.

Garlic:	Helps to lower cholesterol, unblock arteries, and is an antioxidant.
Ginger:	Possesses anti-tumor and anti-inflammatory properties. Also used for morning-sickness, colds, and motion sickness.
Ginkgo Biloba:	Over 50 studies have demonstrated that this herb may boost memory retention, reduce dementia and Alzheimer's.
Ginseng:	Noted for energy boosting and stress relieving effects.
Glucosamine:	Provides relief from osteoarthritis.
Hawthorn:	Used for congestive heart failure. Can be used in teas.
Omega 3 Fatty Acids:	Reduces risk of stroke and heart disease. Also, lubricates joints for arthritis relief.
Saw Palmetto:	Supports healthy prostate functioning, specifically treatment of benign prostate hyperplasia (BPH).
Selenium:	Prevention of various forms of cancer, including prostate, colon, and breast.
Soy Products:	Reduces menopausal symptoms, protects against osteoporosis, and breast cancer, and lowers LDL cholesterol.
St. John's Wort:	Relieves mild depression as effectively as prescription antidepressants without the side effects. It has no effect on severe depression.
Tumeric:	Aches and pains.
Valeran:	Used for insomnia and stress.
Vitamins B, C & E	Keep arteries open.

WARNING: Some of the above supplements are powerful drugs. Do NOT take ANY supplement without medical approval! This is especially important if you're taking medications. For additional information on herbal products you can go to www.herbalgram.org.

CHAPTER TEN:
LIFESTYLE DISEASES CAN KILL YOU!

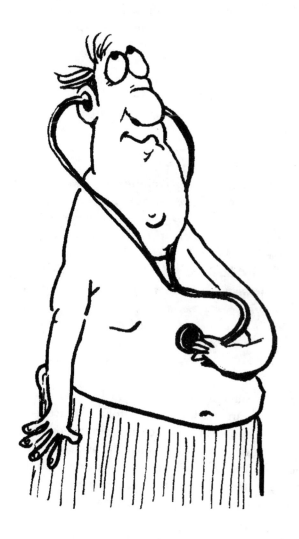

*"Every cigarette you put into your mouth takes 15 minutes off your life!
I don't call them 'cigarettes' anymore, but instead 'cancer-ettes'"*

— Don Alsbro, Founder of Dump Your Plump™

Sixty percent of all deaths in the U.S. are related to heart disease
and cancer ... 80% of these deaths could be prevented.

According to Peter Nielsen, personal trainer to the stars and former Mr. Universe, "You cannot daily pour junk into your stomach, alcohol into your veins, smoke into your lungs, park your butt on the couch and then expect to make a minor course correction somewhere down the line."

Unfortunately, many people have to have a "wakeup call" before they make life changing decisions. It reminds me of the story about the ship and the lighthouse. I'm sure most of you have heard this story, but it bears repeating because there are lighthouses in our paths.

One night at sea, a ship's captain saw what looked like the lights of another ship heading toward him. He had his signalman blink to the other ship, "Change your course 10 degrees south." The reply came back, "Change your course 10 degrees north." The ship's captain answered, "I'm Captain Smith. Change your course south." To which the reply came, "Well, I'm Seaman Jones. Change your course north." This infuriated the captain, so he signaled back, "Damn it, I say change your course south. I'm on a battleship." To which the reply came back, "And I say change your course north. I'm in a lighthouse."

We all have lighthouses in our paths. We can make minor corrections in our ship's path or wait until the heart attack, diabetes, stroke, or cancer occur and try to make a major correction. It reminds me of the truck carrying oil filters for cars that had the slogan painted on the side, "You can pay the price now, or pay later." The big price later is for a new engine (heart attack). There is no such thing as a free lunch! We can't have remotes, three cars, electric garage door openers, 32 ounce "Slurpees," 100 item salad bars and not be willing to pay the small price of activity.

Unfortunately, our Western culture seduces us with no interest in our health. Most of us live to eat, rather than eat to live. As Dr. Hans Diehl of the Lifestyle Medicine Institute, Loma Linda, CA, so often says, "We've worked so hard to have the "good" life and now the "good" life is killing us. However, the good news is that we (you and I) are the determiners of our health and not the doctors. Health is under OUR control."

We should seek the "best" life, not the "good" life. I look at lifestyle diseases as a "hoof and mouth" disease. Most of us do not use our legs for the purpose they were given to us, i.e. walking, running, jumping, and just plain moving around, and we let our mouths, instead of our minds, determine what we eat. We must make the decisions in our head. We are the architects of our health. What kind of a building have you designed and is it proceeding according to plans?

LIFESTYLE DISEASES:
YOU CAN PREVENT THEM!

In reviewing the literature concerning deaths from cardiovascular causes, cancer and diabetes, a commonality runs throughout. A lack of physical activity, excess weight, smoking, high blood pressure, high blood cholesterol, and heredity are the major factors. Of these six factors, YOU control five of them. If you've been reading this

book, you know that all of these risk factors have been thoroughly discussed and that you are pretty much in control of your destiny and that certainly is good news! Genes may load the gun, but YOU choose to pull the trigger!

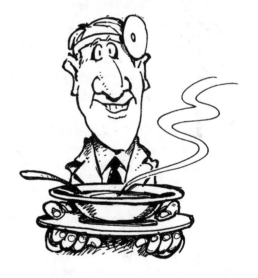

USA Today ran a feature on diabetes and interviewed Ted DeLeon, a Mexican American. He was diagnosed with Type II diabetes (the most common form) nine years ago and has had to learn how to control it through exercise and diet. His parents, aunts and uncles, and seven of nine siblings have it. They all live in the United States. "While genes may set you up for diabetes," he says, "it kicks in when you gain a lot of weight and don't exercise. Where our family ancestors come from in Mexico, they don't have it. Why? They eat beans and tortillas. Meat is a treat. There is no McDonald's. They work a lot (physically), and we don't."

Most medical authorities believe that reducing blood pressure, losing weight, lowering cholesterol and triglycerides, increasing physical activity, and quitting smoking are the most important lifestyle changes you can make if you want to lower your risk for heart disease, cancer, and diabetes.

PREVENTION OF LIFESTYLE DISEASES

Risk Factor	Heart Disease	Diabetes	Cancer
Not maintaining a healthy weight (<25 BMI)	X	X	X
Not exercising 5 days a week (at least 30 minutes)	X	X	X
Smoking	X		X
Not eating a healthy diet (plant-based, low fat)	X	X	X
Drinking alcohol	X	X	X
Not doing prevention (screening, tests)	X	X	X

NOTE: This is not an encompassing list. There are other risk factors such as age, sex, race, and family history that I intentionally did not list. However, according to most experts, preventable factors account for 60% of the causes.

MAJOR CAUSES OF PREMATURE DEATH

Environment	20%
Treatable by Traditional Medicine	10%
Lifestyle Factors	50%
Biological Factors	20%

Healthy People 2000 Report

BOTTOM LINE: The key to avoiding the above diseases is to simply eat a healthy diet, exercise 30 minutes a day, five days a week, refrain from smoke and maintain a healthy body weight. **REMEMBER: YOU CHOOSE TO PULL THE TRIGGER.**

As captain of your ship, become what noted cancer doctor Dr. Bernie Siegel calls a "RESPANT." The word patient means submissive. Dr. Siegel tells his patients not to be patients but to be "respants" – RESponsible particiPANTS in their own health care. Being "respants" means understanding that we are accountable for our actions and inactions. Self-destructive behaviors – drinking, not wearing a seat belt, smoking, eating fast foods, etc. – can't be blamed on society, parents, teachers, or any other outside force.

BE PROACTIVE

"You have the power to maintain your own cardiovascular health. It's up to you to take that responsibility. The choices you make and your habits are much more powerful than anything we in medicine can provide."

— James Rippe, MD Arizona Blue Spring, 2000

Along those same lines, a "respant" helps manage his health by asking the nurse or doctor what his blood pressure, cholesterol, weight, heart rate, temperature, etc. are. I get frustrated when the nurse takes my temperature or resting heart rate and when I ask, "What is it?" She replies, "It's okay." My normal body temperature is 97.5, not 98.6; therefore, when I'm at 98.6 (normal for most), I've actually got a fever. One time I was in the hospital and had a fever of 99.8. The nurse refused to give me medication because her guidelines stated that the temperature had to be 100 degrees before giving fever medication. I had to call the "charge" nurse and threaten to call my doctor before they relented. Knowing your normal temperature or cholesterol is more important than knowing your social security number. **BE A RESPANT!**

BOTTOM LINE: We can choose to practice self-destructive behaviors or we can choose to heal ourselves. **WHAT CHOICES ARE YOU MAKING?**

RESEARCH

We are living in an age in which it has never been easier to obtain health information. Ten years ago you might have gone to a doctor's appointment timidly clutching a newspaper article about your medical condition. Today, it's possible to show up with volumes of information.

The Internet has created a new breed of patient: informed, self confident, and a partner in his/her medical care. There are literally thousands medical internet sites, and they're growing every day. All you have to do is type in the search word, i.e. "cancer" and hundreds of sources will appear. The problem lies in sorting the wheat from the chaff. There are many ways to determine the credibility of the site. A good place to start is with a couple of dependable sites, such as the National Library of Medicine (www.Medlineplus.gov), the National Institute of Health (www.nih.gov), the American Heart Assn. (americanheart.org), the National Cancer Institute (www. cancer.gov), American Diabetes Assn. (www.diabetes.org), and the U.S. Dept. of Health and Human Services (www.healthfinder.gov).

For example, you can evaluate your 10-year risk of heart attack using the Framingham Risk Assesment tool at www.americanheart.org (Click on Diseases, then Risk Assessment). Your score will take into account important risk factors such as total cholesterol, HDL, LDL, triglycerides, blood pressure, and body mass index (BMI).

This is just the tip of the iceberg, but the warning is "buyer beware" (caveat emptor). There are many charlatans out there. On a couple of the web sites mentioned above I mistakenly typed in "com" and not "gov" and got commercial web sites with questionable credentials.

SEARCH OUT THE BEST

Start with your regular doctor, and if he/she accepts you as a PARTNER and you feel that this person is the best choice for this particular problem, then stay there. Otherwise, it may be time to look elsewhere. Talk to friends who have had the same problem. Find out where they received treatment.

Research into the leading medical centers that specialize in treating your illness. When I had my first hip replacement in 1989, I went to Mayo Clinic as I was not comfortable with my local specialists. Except for the inconvenience of getting there and staying in commercial facilities, it doesn't cost any more for treatment there as opposed to medical facilities that do not have the expertise and experience that Mayo has. Now my wife and I feel comfortable with a local orthopedic surgeon so there is no need to travel 500 miles to Mayo's in Rochester, Minnesota.

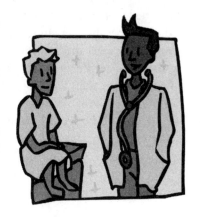

OTHER AVENUES

Integrative or Alternative Medicine. Throughout this book you've read about yoga, acupuncture, Tai Chi, massage, nutrition, meditation, supplementation, spiritualism, physical fitness, and so on. Utilize those resources that will complement your medical treatment. I did NOT say replace your medical treatment.

Spiritual. This will be discussed in greater detail in Chapter 12. There are literally hundreds of medical studies documenting the link between faith and health. A positive spiritual life enhances your mental and physical health, and it even addresses the pain and suffering, as Victor Frankl, survivor of the Nazi death camps, found out. He said, "Suffering ceases to be suffering, once it takes on meaning."

Social Support. Many studies have shown that group support can help people overcome serious diseases. Today, every community has a multitude of support groups. If you can't find one, call your local health department or hospital. In support groups people learn how to improve health habits, how to cope with daily problems and how to express their feelings constructively. You quickly find out that you're not the only one with this problem.

BECOME A RESPANT!
(a RESponsible particiPANT in your own health care)

PROTECTIVE SCREENINGS

The way to cure a medical problem is to stay healthy in the first place. I think we are doing a much better job of that today than we did 20 years ago. More people know their vitals today than they did then, but there is still much more improvement that can be done. Based on your age, sex and risk factors your doctor can give you a schedule for screenings that I call Preventive Maintenance. In the military, "PM" was practiced on your vehicle and other equipment. We change our oil, spark plugs, rotate the tires in our car on a scheduled basis — do our bodies deserve any less? We will have many cars throughout our life — we will only have one body!

There are many screenings. Colonoscopy, digital rectal exam (prostate), total body scans, bone density tests, mammograms, audio and visual screenings.are some of the more common. Following are eight screenings (alphabetical order) that can increase your chances of living a long and healthy life.

RECOMMENDED SCREENINGS

SCREENING TEST	PURPOSE	FREQUENCY OF TEST
Blood Pressure	Detection of heart disease	Whenever possible; if normal, at least once a year
Cholesterol/Triglyceride	Heart/stroke risk	Every 5 years unless levels are high
Fecal Occult	Colon and rectal cancer	Yearly after age 50
Glucose Tolerance	Detect diabetes	Screened annually if risk factors are present
Mammograms	Breast cancer	Annual mammograms after age 40 (women)
Pap Smears	Cervical cancer	After age 18 annually
PSA and digital rectal	Prostate cancer	Annually after age 50 (men)
Sigmoidoscopy	Colon & rectal cancer	Every 5 years after age 50
Colonoscopy	Colon & rectal cancer	Every 10 years after age 50

**CONSULT YOUR DOCTOR ABOUT THE ADVISABILITY
OF THESE TESTS AND OTHERS**

COLON CANCER: THE BEST TEST

Colonoscopy appears to be the most accurate of three tests commonly used to diagnose colon cancer, the country's second leading cancer killer. In a recent study, 2,885 men ages 50 - 75 with no signs of colon cancer were screened with a fecal occult-blood test, using stool samples collected over three days, and a sigmoidoscopy in which the lower third of the colon is viewed with a flexible tube. Then the men had a colonoscopy to view the entire intestine.

The blood text and the sigmoidoscopy missed 24 percent of tumors and over 280 precancerous growths that were found by the colonoscopy. Many doctors recommend a colonoscopy at age 50, then at 10 or 15 year intervals if nothing is found. (New England Journal of Medicine)

HEALTH BY THE NUMBERS:

RISK FACTOR	READINGS			
Glucose	Normal:	<100		
(fasting plasma)	Impaired:	100-125		
	Diabetes:	128+		

Blood Pressure		Systolic		Diastolic
	Optimal:	115	and	75
	Normal:	<120	and	<80
	Prehypertension:	120-139	or	80-90
	Hypertension:	140+	or	90+

Cholesterol Total:	Desirable:	<200
	Borderline High:	200-239
	High:	240+

LDL	Optimal:	<100
	Near/Above Optimal:	100-129
	Borderline High:	160-189
	High:	190+

HDL:	Low:	<40
	High:	60+

Diabetes occurs when the body either doesn't produce enough insulin (Type I) or the cells become resistant to the insulin being produced (Type II). Insulin is a form of blood glucose that is used by the body for fuel. Think of insulin as a "delivery" truck that goes from the pancreas to the cells and back, with each cell having a gate keeper. In the normal cell, the gate keeper opens the cell to receive the energy, and everything is fine. However, in Type I diabetes (only about 5%), the delivery truck never arrives. Therefore, the insulin must be delivered in the form of an injection.

In Type II (used to be called adult onset-but we are finding it in young children), the delivery truck delivers the cargo (insulin), but either it is not enough (usually because of being overweight), or the gate keeper refuses to open the cell. One way to view it is the delivery man rings the doorbell, but no one is there to open the door. The solution isn't to make more insulin, but to make the gates work better.

The American Diabetes Association (ADA – 800-342-2383 or www.diabetes.org) estimates that about 18.2 million people in the U.S. have diabetes. Pevalence of the disease has increased nearly 50 % in the past decade; the rise is directly linked to the 60 percent increase in obesity over the same period. John Buse, MD, of the University of North Carolina School of Medicine, says "the worst-case scenario is that we'll just get fatter and fatter and more sedentary until we all look like Jabba the Hutt (the obese crime kingpin from Star Wars) and everyone will have diabetes in the 40's and 50's."

Diabetes is NOT a sugar problem. It is a FAT problem. Excess fat intake is a key factor in decreasing and inactivating insulin receptors (gate keepers). Studies have repeatedly shown that by changing the diet to that of simple foods, i.e. fruits and vegetables and losing a few pounds of weight, that a majority of Type II diabetics can be off insulin within weeks.

CHOICE:

a. Stay on a high fat, high sugar diet, and take pills/shots. OR
b. Eat a simple diet of grains, fruits, and vegetables and not have to take pills/shots.

WHICH DO YOU CHOOSE?

NOTE:
**DO NOT MAKE CHANGES IN YOUR PRESCRIBED INSULIN LEVELS
WITHOUT FIRST CONSULTING A PHYSICIAN.**

WHAT ARE THE RED FLAGS FOR DIABETES?

TYPE I (insulin dependent):
Excessive thirst
Extreme hunger
Increased urination
Unexplained weight loss

TYPE II (non-insulin dependent)
All of the symptoms for Type I
Blurry vision
Frequent skin and bladder infections
Slow-healing wounds
Tingling or numbness in extremities

We need to start living "the good life" NOW! Later should not be an option! Most authorities agree that approximately 60% of all deaths in the U.S. are related to lifestyle factors and that 80% of these deaths could be prevented. According to the Surgeon General's Report on Health Promotion and Disease Prevention, "Americans annually lose 15 million years of living from preventable causes.

SIMPLIFIED TYPE 2 DIABETES EXPLANATION

TWO SCENARIOS:

1. Key (Insulin) won't open the door (body cell)
2. Delivery truck (bloodstream) can't deliver its cargo (insulin) because of failure by the manufacturer (pancreas) to make enough.

       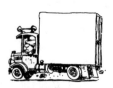   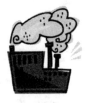

BODY   BLOODSTREAM   INSULIN   PANCREAS

OSTEOPOROSIS MYTHS

MYTH: We need to increase our intake of calcium.

FACT: For this myth I would like to borrow the expertise of Dr. Hans Diehl, developer of the Coronary Health Improvement Program (CHIP). He contends that everyone knows that you can't save money when you spend more than you make. This is what happens to the calcium in our bodies. Because of our Western diet of animal protein, whole dairy products, salt, phosphoric acid (soda) and caffeine, the body "spends" an extraordinary amount of calcium to process these foods. When there is not enough calcium available in the diet, it "borrows" from another source-the bones. Slowly over the years this leeching process causes the bones to become brittle and weak.

I spent two years in Vietnam and never saw a case of osteoporosis, despite the fact that their calcium intake is as little as 300 mg a day (1/5 of what U.S. government agencies recommend for American women). The Vietnamese don't even have the word, osteoporosis, in their language.

MYTH: The best prevention for osteoporosis is a calcium supplement

FACT: This goes along with the previous myth. It's strangely paradoxical that osteoporosis has become epidemic in the U.S. where the consumption of calcium-rich dairy products and calcium supplements is the highest in the world. Americans eat 2-3 times more protein than they need. This high intake requires a voluminous amount of calcium, more than we can get from a supplement or from food. As stated above, the body will steal calcium from your bones to get what it needs elsewhere.

MYTH: I'm too young to be concerned about my bone health

FACT: By the time you're 25-30 years old, you've reached your peak bone mass. At this point you can't add more bone mass, but you can keep your "bone bank" from being depleted by changing your diet and exercising.

MYTH: Any kind of exercise is good for the bones.

FACT: Not all types of aerobic activity are equally good for warding off osteoporosis. The top choices are: hiking, jogging, fitness walking, weight training, racquetball, tennis, volleyball, basketball and jump rope. In other words, weight bearing exercises are best.

THE ANSWER TO ALL OF THESE MYTHS IS TO REDUCE OUR PROTEIN INTAKE, DO WEIGHT BEARING EXERCISE, AND HAVE A HEALTHY DIET LOW IN SALT, FAT, PHOSPHORIC ACID, AND CAFFEINE.

If you have concerns about Osteoporosis, you need to talk to your physician. Post-menopausal women need to have a bone density test. There are several new drugs on the market that show promise in slowing and stopping bone loss and even promoting new bone growth.

HEART DISEASE: YOU CAN PREVENT IT!

In the early part of this book, you learned that excess weight contributes to heart disease, the NUMBER ONE killer in America. Fifty percent (one out of two) of us will die from cardiovascular disease. So while I have your attention, it seems a good time to heighten your awareness of the risk factors for heart disease.

Risk Factors for Heart Disease:

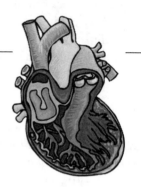

1. High blood pressure
2. Elevated blood cholesterol and/or triglycerides
3. Smoking
4. Excess body weight
5. Diabetes (Adult onset, Type II)
6. Lack of physical activity
7. Family history (heredity)
8. Age
9. Gender (until menopause, males have a higher risk)
10. Race

OF THESE TEN FACTORS, YOU CONTROL THE FIRST SIX.

Most medical authorities believe that reducing blood pressure, increasing physical activity, and quitting smoking are the three most important lifestyle changes you should make, if you want to lower your risk for heart disease. Your participation in an exercise program is a significant first step toward lowering your risk. In addition, many participants find that as they increase their physical activity and decrease body fat, their doctor may be able to decrease or even stop their medications.

> # NEVER STOP TAKING PRESCRIBED MEDICATION UNLESS YOU'VE OBTAINED THE PERMISSION OF YOUR PHYSICIAN!

BLOOD PRESSURE

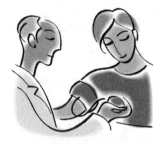

BLOOD PRESSURE RANGES	
OPTIMAL	115/76
NORMAL	120/80
HIGH-NORMAL	≤139/89
HIGH	≥140/90

JNCPD 6th report, NIH

Question: What do these numbers mean?

SYSTOLIC (the top number) is the pressure placed on your arteries while the heart is contracting and pumping blood.

DIASTOLIC (the bottom number) is the arterial pressure between beats.
What is Your Blood Pressure? _____

What YOU can do about high blood pressure.

• **LOSE WEIGHT IF YOU'RE OVERWEIGHT.** Of all the non-drug methods of hypertension control, this is the most effective.

• **EXERCISE REGULARLY.** Regular aerobic exercise, at least 3-4 times a week for 15-30 minutes, can reduce hypertension as much as 20%.

• **REDUCE YOUR SALT INTAKE.** Most of us consume 2-3 times more salt than we need. If you can reduce the intake to under 1,600 mg, it will help. In addition, take the salt shakers off the table and read labels of all packaged food closely for salt content.

• **DRINK LESS ALCOHOL.** If you have high blood pressure, it is vital that you control your alcohol intake to less than two drinks a day.

• **QUIT SMOKING.** Smoking causes the smoker to have a risk 2-3 times higher than non smokers.

• **EAT LESS FAT.** A low fat diet lowers cholesterol and blood pressure.

Are You Salt Sensitive?

About 1/3 of American people are salt sensitive. This causes the body to retain excess water in the bloodstream, thus raising blood pressure AND weight. To determine if you're salt sensitive, get your blood pressure measured while on your normal diet, and then restrict salt for a couple of months and have it taken again. Be sure that the only change you make is dietary.

If you want a low sodium diet, try the DASH diet (Dietary Approaches to Stop Hypertension) at www.nhlbi.nih.gov/health/public/heart/hbp/dash/new_dash.pdf.

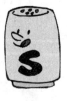

IMPACT OF LIFESTYLE MODIFICATIONS ON BLOOD PRESSURE (BP)	
RECOMMENDATION	**BP REDUCTION**
Maintain ideal body weight	5-20 mmHg
Low fat, high fruit & vegetable diet	8-14 mmHg
Sodium intake ≤2.4 grams per day	2-8 mmHg
Exercise at least 30 minutes most days	4-9 mmHg
Limit alcohol intake (men ≤2; women ≤1 drink)	2-4 mmHg

University Medical Specialties, Berrien Springs, MI

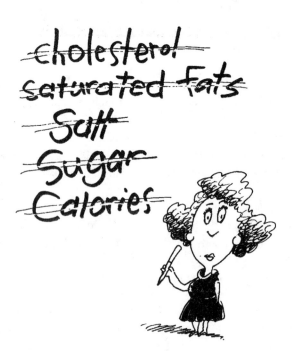

ADDITIONAL LIFESTYLE MODIFICATIONS FOR HEALTHY BLOOD PRESSURE

- Know your cholesterol level. If it's high, modify your diet, and if that's unsuccessful, ask your doctor for medication.

- Have your blood pressure checked every six months and monthly if it's high.

- Ask your doctor whether you have irregular heartbeats or circulation problems that can be controlled through aspirin or other blood thinning medication.

- If you're diabetic, follow your doctor's recommendations for keeping your condition under control.

- If you experience any stroke symptoms such as sudden weakness or numbness in your face, arm or leg; blurred or decreased vision; dizziness or loss of coordination – seek immediate medical attention.

- Practice meditation or relaxation techniques. Practicing the "relaxation response" outlined by Dr. Herbert Benson in The Wellness Book, for 10-15 minutes daily can reduce blood pressure 10-15% (and cholesterol also). (Benson)

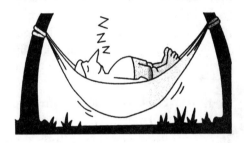

Meditation for Beginners: The Do Nothing Technique

TIME: 3-5 minutes
POSTURE: Lying down or sitting
WHEN: Anytime

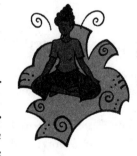

Sit or lie down and just allow your mind to do its thing. Your aim is to be there without trying to control. Let your attention go anywhere it wants. You can think about sex, your to-do lists, movies, nothing, or everything. Notice where your mind goes. This exercise helps you overcome the notion that the human mind has to be controlled, even when you are resting. You want to be in the same state you're in when you are about to fall asleep. Just let the mind drift. You are intentionally doing nothing. You cannot fail.

STROKES, HEART ATTACKS AND CHOKING

STROKES

A man's last years ought to be spent strapped to the fighting chair of a game fisher while battling a black marlin, not tethered to a nursing home — in bed, incontinent, and unable to talk. The latter is a likely scenario if you're one of the 700,000 who will have a stroke this year. While 25 percent will die, 40 % will be disabled, many severely.

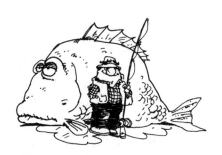

Strokes are the third leading cause of death in the U.S. (behind heart attack and cancer). Eighty percent of strokes are ischemic strokes that involve a blood clot. In fact, a stroke is just like a heart attack, only instead of heart cells dying for lack of blood, brain cells are dying. This is why it's been termed a "brain attack."

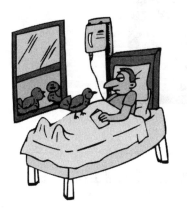

Strokes can be prevented with a lifestyle similar to the prevention of heart disease. Change to plant based diet, lower stress, do daily aerobic activity, lift weights at least two times a week, practice meditation, follow a medication plan prescribed by your physician, and look at implementing a supplementation program.

ONE MINUTE STROKE TEST

Would you be willing to spend one minute to save a person from the ravages of a stroke? A quick amateur diagnosis and call for emergency help will greatly reduce the chances of paralysis, speech impairments, and other disabilities. A major NIH study found that patients who got a clot-busting drug within three hours of the FIRST symptoms stood a better chance of avoiding disability.

CINCINNATI STROKE SCALE TEST (FAS)

This test can be done in one minute, by people with no medical training and is very accurate in its diagnosis. It involves tests for:

Facial droop:	Normal:	Both sides of the face move equally.
	Abnormal:	One side of the face does not move at all.
Arm drift:	Normal:	Both arms move equally or not at all.
	Abnormal:	One arm drifts compared to the other.
Speech:	Normal:	Person uses correct words with no slurring.
	Abnormal:	Slurred or inappropriate words or mute.

TO PERFORM THE FAS TEST: *Ask the individual to smile or fake a smile, move their arms, and speak a sentence. If the results seem abnormal, CALL 911!*

CHOKING

Your dinner companion can't breathe, can't talk and is turning blue. He is gasping for air and puts his hand to his throat. These signs tell you he is choking. Do you know what to do?

Choking is an emergency that cannot wait for the emergency room. In most cases the victims fate will be decided by the time emergency personnel arrive. Either a knowledgeable person steps forward and relieves the choking or there's a good chance the person won't survive.

UNIVERSAL CHOKING SIGN

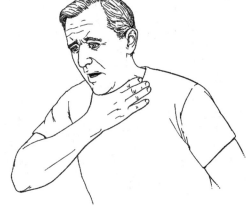

HEIMLICH MANEUVER

You can be that knowledgeable person by using the Heimlich maneuver or abdominal thrust. Here's how you do it:

- Stand behind the choking person and wrap your arms around his waist.

- Make a fist with one hand. Place the thumb side of you fist against the person's abdomen, just above the navel, but well below the sternum..

- Grasp your fist with the other hand.

- Give a quick upward thrust into the abdomen.

- Repeat until the object pops out or the person loses consciousness.

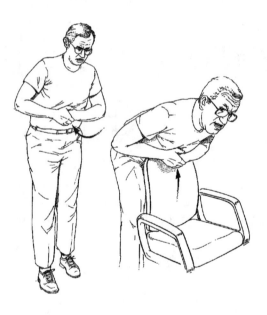

SELF HEIMLICH:
Do abdominal thrusts on yourself or lean over the back of a chair and press forcefully.

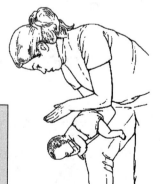

WARNINGS:

- Do not use the Heimlich if the person can talk.
- Use less force for a child.

THE "NEW" CPR

Seattle WA. A city famous for saving cardiac victims, has discovered that telling frantic 911 callers how to perform mouth to mouth resuscitation resulted in less lives saved.

In the first moments of a cardiac arrest, help usually comes from a bystander who is reluctant or doesn't know how to perform mouth to mouth resuscitation. The window of opportunity for life is six minutes. That is how long rescuers have to get the heart started for the victim to survive. It usually takes longer than this for 911 personnel to arrive.

The goal is to get the chest compressions started immediately and keep the compressions going until trained rescuers arrive. Research has shown that blood in the body still has the oxygen that was picked by when it last passed through the lungs before the heart stopped. The body needs the chest compressions to keep the blood moving.

PERFORMING CHEST COMPRESSIONS

Place the heel of your hand on the breastbone in the center of the chest. Place the other hand on top of the hand, intertwining the fingers. Keeping the elbows locked and arms straight, push down firmly compressing the chest 2". Only the heel of the hand touches the chest. Release. Continue uninterrupted at the rate of 100 compressions per minute until help arrives.

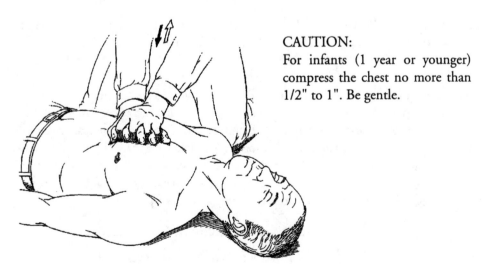

CAUTION:
For infants (1 year or younger) compress the chest no more than 1/2" to 1". Be gentle.

TRIGLYCERIDES

Triglycerides are fats that circulate in the bloodstream. Levels are usually taken after an overnight fast at the same time cholesterol levels are analyzed. The average fasting triglycerides level is 120-125 mg/dl. Levels above 200 mg/dl are associated with arterial aging. According to the "Real Age" program, a triglycerides level of 210 for a male age 55 translates into a body age of 60.9 (5.9 added years).

TRIGLYCERIDES AND CHOLESTEROL: WHAT'S NORMAL, WHAT'S NOT		
High Risk Level	**Desirable Level**	**Borderline Level**
LDL - 161 and higher	Up to 129*	130 to 160
HDL - 39 and lower	50 and higher	40 to 49
Trigly - 401 and higher	Up to 199	200 to 400
Total chol - 241 and higher	Up to 199*	200 to 240

If you have coronary disease or multiple coronary risk factors, desirable LDL should be 100 or lower and total cholesterol below 150. National Cholesterol Education program, 2001 report.

CHOLESTEROL: WHAT YOU DON'T KNOW CAN KILL YOU!

Many people don't realize that cholesterol is only in animal products, i.e. meat, eggs, and dairy products. However, even more dangerous than cholesterol is saturated fat (found in both animal and plant foods).

Saturated fat (which is different from cholesterol itself) has a greater effect on elevating blood cholesterol and contributing to heart disease. In fact, according to Dr. William Castelli, director of the famous 50 year old Framingham, Massachusetts project, saturated fats are four times more harmful in raising blood cholesterol than dietary cholesterol itself. Saturated fats are the major ingredients in many packaged foods and commercial baked goods. They are also in nondairy creamers, candy bars, butter, eggnog, ice cream, cheese, egg yolks, liver, steak, fried foods, creams, sauces, and gravies.

Cholesterol is only in animal products

Scientific studies show that people with high blood cholesterol are more likely to develop coronary heart disease. This risk increases in direct proportion to the elevation of the cholesterol. For example, people with total blood cholesterol readings higher than 265 have four times the risk of developing heart disease as those with levels of 190 or lower. Since every 1% decrease in blood cholesterol means a 2% decrease in the risk of heart disease, you want to use these cholesterol elevating products sparingly.

A one percent decrease in blood cholesterol means a two percent decrease in the risk of heart disease.

BLOOD CHOLESTEROL RATIOS

CHOLESTEROL RATIOS: Many authorities believe that the cholesterol ratio numbers are even more important indicators of heart disease than the individual cholesterol numbers. The ratios help tell us whether more cholesterol is being stored in our cells (bad) or else is being broken down and removed from our body (good). To determine these ratios for yourself, simply divide your total cholesterol and LDL numbers by your HDL number.

	PROTECTIVE	WARNING
Total Chol/HDL	Less than 4.2	4.3 and higher
LDL/HDL	Less than 2.5	2.6 and higher

What is your Total Cholesterol/HDL ratio? $\dfrac{\text{Total Chol}}{\text{HDL}}$ = _____

What is your LDL/HDL ratio? $\dfrac{\text{LDL}}{\text{HDL}}$ = _____

THREE PLANS TO FAT-PROOF YOUR HEART

Plan 1: Lowering LDL (Bad) Cholesterol:

Concentrate on banning SATURATED and Trans-fats. To determine your level of 10% or less from saturated fat, multiply the number of calories you eat (the average man consumes 2,500 a day) by .1, and divide the result (250 in this example) by 9 (number of calories in one gram of fat.). For this example, the 28 g of saturated fat is the fat threshold for a 2,500 calorie diet. If you are trying to stay under 25% total fat for the day, multiply the saturated fat limit (28 g) by 2.5. So 70 g or 630 calories would be the total fat limit for a 2,500 calorie diet.

1. Choose oatmeal. In a study, it was found that by eating oat bran or oatmeal daily for six weeks, without any other dietary changes, LDL was reduced 10-16%.

2. Drop a dress/suit size. By dropping just 5-10 lbs, you can maintain your HDL level and double the LDL reduction.

3. Manage your anger. Men who deal with stress calmly had LDL levels 10% lower than those who lashed out or suppressed their feelings.

WHAT IS YOUR LDL? _____

Plan 2: Raising HDL (Good) Cholesterol

1. Work up a sweat. Aerobic exercise (at least 3 times a week for 45 minutes) increases the HDL levels 11-19% higher than being inactive.

2. Throw away the "cigarette." Smoking depresses the HDL about 6% according to 54 studies in the British Medical Journal.

3. Have an orange. Getting the daily 60 mg of Vitamin C can increase the HDL level about 10%.

WHAT IS YOUR HDL? _____

Plan 3: Lowering Triglycerides

1. Go fishing. Eating more cold water fish, especially tuna, salmon and lake trout can significantly reduce the tri's. One reason for this is that they contain omega 3 fatty acids which inhibit the liver's production of triglycerides.

> **OMEGA-3:** *Omega-3 fats (polyunsaturated fatty acids often referred to as "good fats") are some of the most potent nutrients for heart health. These essential fats, found primarily in seafood, but also in flaxseed oil, not only lower your risk of heart disease, but may also stave off a number of age-related diseases including Alzheimer's. Studies indicate that eating as little as 1-2 servings a week of omega-3 fatty acids can greatly reduce the risk of heart disease. Sources of omega-3 are salmon, trout, tuna, mackerel, herring, sardines, and fish oil capsules.*

2. Hit the gym. Working out and eating a diet low in saturated fat can reduce triglycerides by as much as 50%.

WHAT IS YOUR TRIGLYCERIDE LEVEL? _____

DO YOU NEED THE NEW HEART TESTS?

Is Cholesterol the Entire Story?

Your cholesterol test came back and your LDL was under 89, your HDL was over 50 and your total cholesterol was 139. Do you need another test? Several years ago, I was in that situation, and, even with those supposedly "good" numbers, I suffered a heart attack. I have since discovered that I wasn't an exception. Over half of all people who suffer heart attacks have normal cholesterol levels. Unfortunately, I learned too late that I had elevated levels of C-reactive protein (CRP) and homocysteine.

C - REACTIVE PROTEIN (CRP)

It has recently been discovered that C-reactive protein and homocysteine play a much bigger role than previously thought in causing heart disease. In the 60's a Harvard pathologist discovered these risk factors and tried to get them into mainstream medicine. However, he failed, and consequently 30 years later we are finding out that these two markers are very significant. There have been 22 studies that show CRP is a strong independent risk factor for heart disease.

Both of these markers are indicators of inflammation in the blood vessel walls. A large study of 28,000 women over an eight year period found that for some people, the CRP test was a better predictor of who would have a heart attack than cholesterol readings. As a matter of fact, the increase in risk for heart disease was over 300%. Elevated CRP also raised the risks for diabetes, stroke, cancer, and Alzheimer's.

A CRP reading of 3 mg per liter or higher is considered to be elevated. The good news is that if you have this factor there are several treatment options. First off, exercising and losing weight can lower the CRP levels, as well as the "statin" drugs that are used to treat elevated cholesterol. The CRP test costs about $25 and, in many cases, is covered by insurance if done for diagnostic purposes.

HOMOCYSTEINE

Homocysteine is another marker for inflammation. In high levels, homocysteine is thought to give LDL a helping hand in promoting hardening of the arteries. A high level is considered to be 10 or higher mg-per liter, and again this is another relatively inexpensive test. While high-protein animal foods raise homocysteine levels, a diet of plant-based foods and supplements of B6, B12, folate (folic acid) and the amino acid N-acetyl-cystein (NAC) can help lower the level. Supplements are essential, as folic acid is not well absorbed from food. For the exact supplement formula, you need, you should see medical personnel that are knowledgeable in supplementation.

LOWERING HOMOCYSTEINE	
B6	50 mg
B12	100 mg
Folate	1,000 mcg
NAC	1,800 mg

Dr. Seth Baum, MD
Medical Director of the
Mind/Body Medical Institute

CANCER

YOUR "CANCERETTES" OR YOUR HEALTH
(THE CHOICE IS YOURS)

According to Dr. Roizen, the author of "Real Age," if you're a smoker and have a pack-a-day habit, you add eight years to your actual age. If you're forty, how does forty-eight sound? Even if you don't smoke, but live with a smoker or work in a smoke-filled environment just four hours a day, can add seven years to your actual age.

Every year, 500,000 Americans die from cigarette smoking. That huge number doesn't include the countless others who suffer from lung disease, stroke, hearing loss, impaired vision, and osteoporosis. Smoking also damages the immune system, the neurological system, the ears, nose, and throat, the digestive system, and MORE!

> *Every cigarette you put in your mouth takes 15 minutes off your life! That's the bad news. The good news is that you have a choice.*

Every cigarette you put in your mouth takes 15 minutes off your life! I don't call them cigarettes anymore, but "cancerettes" because that is what they're designed to produce. If you don't die from something else first, you'll die from a smoking related disease. What is even sadder, is that, for many, it isn't the dying that is the tragedy, but the quality of life that precedes the death. Have you ever watched a person die of emphysema? When I was eight years, old I watched my father die prematurely of a heart attack related to "cancerettes," and when I was sixteen, I saw my best friend's father suffer for three years and go from 180 lbs to 100 before dying of emphysema. "Cancerettes" are designed to kill!

That's the bad news. The good news is that you have a choice. Every "cancerette" you smoke is your choice to get older faster and every "cancerette" you don't smoke is a choice to get younger. If you're a pack-a-day smoker, and you stop smoking today, within five years, you can save seven of those years. That means that by making a choice to stop when you're 40 years old, that by the time you're 45 years old, your body will think it's only 46 years old, instead of 53. By making some of the other changes, such as eating better and exercising, you could have the body of a 33 year old. Just think, the difference of 20 years just by doing some simple common sense prevention.

Web Sites For Cancer Information:
National Cancer Institute: www.cancer.gov
American Cancer Society: www.cancer.org

CONSIDER QUITTING.

If you or a friend are ready to consider quitting (remember, it is the smoker who must want to quit, not the friend), then do the following:

a. Revisit your earlier decisions to quit smoking and make a list of your failed attempts and the reasons for the failures.

b. Make a list of all the cues that trigger your impulse to light up and write down how to avoid those cues.

c. Pick a "quit" day, preferably within a week of when you complete the above lists and mark it on all your calendars, mirrors, and tell your SUPPORTIVE friends.

QUIT! It will be the best single thing you've ever done for your body AND your loved ones.

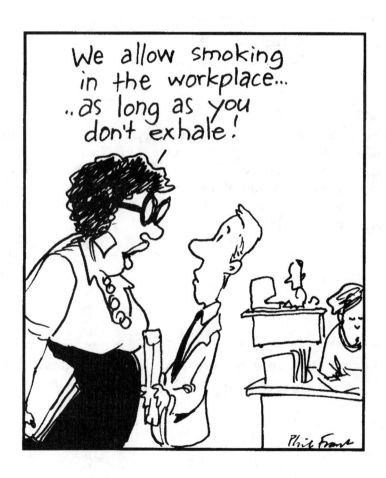

IT'S ALL IN THE FAMILY

"My name is Patrick Reynolds. My grandfather, R.J. Reynolds, founded the tobacco company that makes Camels, Winstons, and Salems. We've all heard the tobacco industry say smoking doesn't cause health problems. Well, they ought to look at the R.J. Reynolds family tree.

- My grandfather chewed tobacco and died of cancer.
- My father smoked heavily and died of emphysema.
- My mother smoked and had emphysema and heart disease.
- My two aunts, also heavy smokers, died of emphysema and cancer.
- Currently, three of my older brothers who smoke have emphysema.
- I smoked for 10 years and now have something called 'small airways lung disease.'

Do you really think the tobacco companies are being truthful?"

— Patrick Reynolds, Public Service Ad

The two chief by-products of cancer-ettes – nicotine and carbon monoxide – work together to increase the strain on the heart. Nicotine is a stimulant, causing the heart to beat faster. Therefore, the heart needs more oxygen to support its higher rate of activity. However, the carbon monoxide absorbs the oxygen, reducing the amount available to the heart, thus placing a strain on the cardiac muscle.

BOTTOM LINE:

The strain of smoking one pack of cancer-ettes a day is equal to being 100 lbs. overweight!!!

COLON CANCER

After lung cancer, colon cancer is the biggest cancer killer of Americans. As you can see below, there are many lifestyle steps you can take to reduce your risk.

BEST BETS FOR PREVENTING COLON CANCER:

1. Avoid a high-fat diet

2. Eat lots of vegetables, fruits and whole grains

3. Exercise regularly and avoid excess calories. Obesity increases your risk

4. Get enough Folic Acid (B vitamin) — at least 400 mcg a day

5. Avoid charbroiled and fried foods

6. Don't smoke

7. Get screened — it can save your life. Fecal occult tests, colonoscopies and sigmoidoscopies should be started at age 50 (earlier if there are significant risk factors).

By the time symptoms appear the disease is often advanced. According to the Center for Disease Control, up to 90% of the cases could be avoided by screening. Nearly 75% of colon cancers occur in people over 50 who have none of the above risk factors.

CANCER CLINICAL TRIALS

Many people claim that clinical trials are cancer research's best kept secret, and that if people knew about it, as many as 100,000 who die of cancer each year could be saved. According to the National Cancer Institute in Bethesda, Maryland, "If all patients with cancer were treated in the context of clinical trials, cancer mortality would drop 10%."

For example, according to the American Cancer Society (www.cancer.org), in April 2002, there were over 400 new drugs ready for entry into clinical trials, (a necessary procedure for FDA approval), but because so few patients are available, only about 100 would be able to be tested.

> **REAL MEN SEE DOCTORS**
>
> *A man has a 1 in 2 lifetime chance of developing cancer, compared with a woman's 1 in 3 chance.*
>
> *(AARP Bulletin 16)*

To receive more information on this option, call the National Cancer Institute to get general information and then talk to your physician about being a participant. To learn about the 5,000+ clinical research studies sponsored by the National Institute of Health, go to www.ClinicalTrials.gov. Another reliable source to learn about trials, drug information, and the latest on a disease is the National Library of Medicine. (Medlineplus.gov or 1-888-FIND-NLM).

DETER AND PROTECT

In the previous chapter I discussed supplementation and its uses in the prevention of chronic diseases. Research is continually being done to determine if diseases can be significantly affected by over-the-counter and prescription medicine or nutritional supplements.

Keeping up on the latest research results on all preventative measures is your best medicine. As of Jan. 2004, the current research indicates that certain supplements may lower your risk of chronic diseases.

TAKING THIS:	MAY LOWER YOUR RISK OF:
Calcium, Vitamin D	Osteoporosis & Colon Cancer
Aspirin, Statins, Antibiotics, Omega-3 fatty acids, folic acid	Heart Disease & Stroke
Aspirin, Statins, Ginkgo Biloba	Dementia
Aspirin, Celecoxib	Colon Cancer
Finasteride, Vitamin E, Selenium, Saw Palmetto	Prostate Cancer
Trtinoin	Skin Cancer
Celecoxib	Lung Cancer
Oral Contraceptives	Ovarian Cancer
Tamoxifen, Raloxifene, Aromatase, Inhibitors	Breast Cancer

It appears that we are on the verge of developing a pill that will help fight obesity, quit smoking, ease arterial inflammation and raise HDL (good) cholesterol. What a pill!

James Cleeman of the National Heart, Lung and Blood Institute says that there is "an unquenchable desire in the national psyche to find a magic bullet that will solve our problem. However, a pill can't mimic the benefits of a healthy diet, exercise and not smoking."

Richard Milani, MD, head of Cardiac Prevention and Rehabilitation at the Ochsner Clinic in New Orleans, puts it more bluntly. "It's just goofy that we have to come up with concoctions to take care of our poor behaviors. Look what it is we're spending our resources to undo. We got here for a good reason. There's no such thing as a sudden heart attack. It takes years of preparation."

Art Caplan, a bioethicist at the University of Pennsylvania, said the emphasis on drugs shifts responsibility from the individual, the food industry, and society at large to the medical profession. "People love to find a quick fix. They can say, 'Oh well, I'm not indulgent, I'm just sick.' We are in love with the idea that medicine can bail us out of all kinds of woes, ailments and problems. And, even though we complain the costs are killing us, we can't stop."

BOTTOM LINE:

Damage to the body can't be undone and eventually risky behaviors take their toll. There is no such thing as a free lunch, i.e. eat "bad" foods, be inactive, smoke and then take a pill to make it go away!

Cancer, heart disease, diabetes, and other diseases develop because of heredity, which you can't control; and lifestyle, which you CAN control. Don't smoke, stay at optimum weight, eat a plant-based diet with lots of fruits, vegetables, beans, whole grains, and a minimum of meat. Limit consumption of saturated fat. Drink moderately, if at all. AND get REGULAR exercise.

GOOD LUCK!
I KNOW YOU CAN DO IT!!

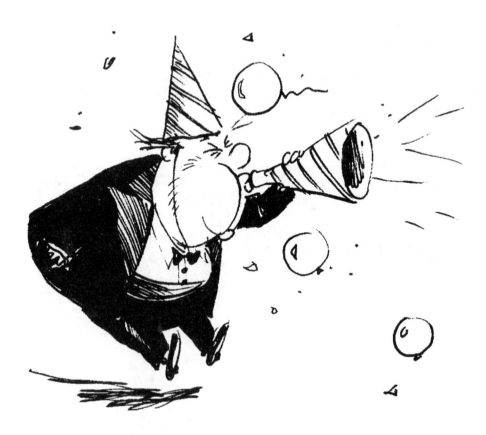

CHAPTER ELEVEN:
STRESS: A SILENT KILLER

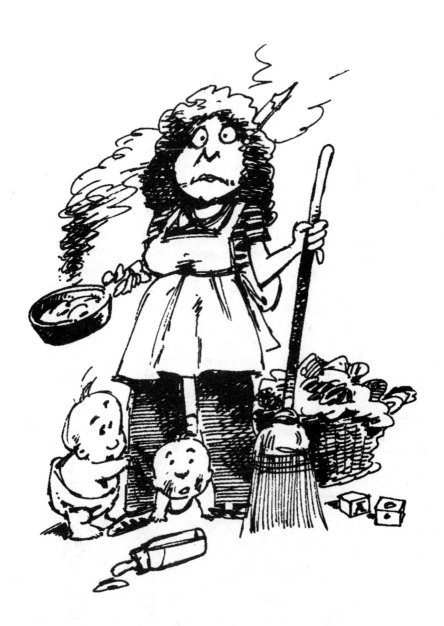

STRESSED?

SERENITY PRAYER

"Lord, give me the courage to change the things I can, the serenity to accept the things that I can't change and the wisdom to know the difference."

— Rheinhold Neibuhr

INTRODUCTION

When I finished writing "The Best Little Book of Wellness," I realized that I couldn't truthfully say it was the "best little book" because it did not have chapters on stress and spirituality. After all, you can't separate the mind, body and spirit.

I knew that I was going to be in Sedona, Arizona for a couple of weeks and that this would be the perfect place to write a chapter on stress. Talk about paradise. There is something about the peace and tranquility of the red rocks that everyone should experience at least once in their lifetime. Maybe for you it would be the ocean, or a mountain stream. The important thing is that everyone should have a place to go where they, feel peace and tranquillity.

Few people could be stressed in an environment like this, and throughout the upcoming year, I will take frequent 10-15 minute mini vacations and recall the peace that I felt in the "Red Rock" country. I have a screen saver on my computer of 150 Sedona scenes so that I'm never far away from the rocks. My good friend Paul has a cottage on a lake in northern Wisconsin. He put a digital picture of himself fishing at sunset on his computer as a screen-saver and that is his stress reliever.

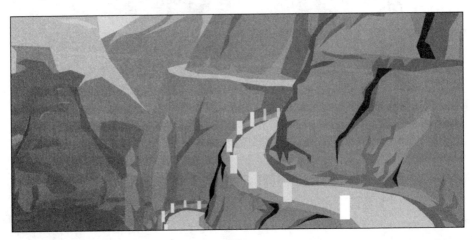

WHAT IS STRESS?

DEFINITION OF STRESS: Hans Selye, noted psychiatrist, defined stress as the "nonspecific response of the body to any demand on it." Nonspecific means that the body goes through a number of intense, biochemical reactions and re-adjustments without regard to the nature of the stress causing event. In general terms, stress is anything that you interpret as a threat to your stability or equilibrium.

There are positive and negative aspects of stress. The negative aspect is that stress triggers the adaptive functions directed at establishing normal psychological states. One effect of this adaptive function over a long period of time can be "distress" which is characterized by tension, insecurity, and frustrations. Untreated distress can lead to a variety of illnesses such as headaches, ulcers, high blood pressure, and even suicide.

This is the negative side of stress. The positive side is that stress can be enjoyed and is considered an essential element of life. Without stress, most of the technological advances that we enjoy today would never have been discovered. We must accept that stress is inevitable, desirable, but potentially harmful. The key is learning to manage it and not let it manage us. If we aren't prepared, then the results could cause distress, tension and a generally reduced quality of life. NEVER LET STRESS AFFECT YOUR VALUE SYSTEM!

STRESSORS

In order to have stress, we must have stressors. A stressor is a stimulus with the POTENTIAL of triggering bodily reactions: We all have stressors in our lives: situations, people, or things which we must adapt to. Stressors can be too much work or not enough time to do the job, the pressure of making good grades in school, the desire to make new friends, and our own traits such as being quick to anger, shy, conscious about weight, etc. Although these are stressors, it doesn't necessarily mean that we're stressed. It only means that they have the potential to produce the stress response.

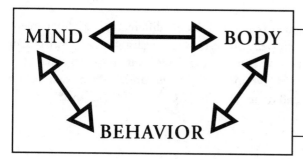

This illustration is designed to show the inter-connectiveness of stress.

Stressors come in many forms:

- Biological — toxins that cause disease, heat or cold in the body.
- Psychological — threats to our self esteem that cause depression.
- Sociological — death of a loved one, divorce or separation, loss of a job.
- Time — not having enough.
- Philosophical — our purpose in life.

STRESS MODEL

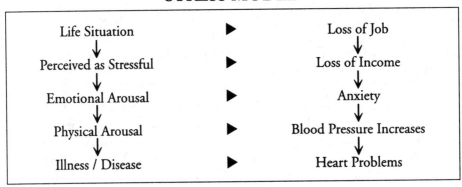

BOTTOM LINE: Stress is our subjective response to a situation.
YOU HAVE THE POWER to control your own stress response.
YOU HAVE THE POWER to stop this chain of events at any stage.

FEAR AS A STRESSOR

We all know that fear can be a major stressor. I will not be able to do justice to this topic in these few paragraphs, but if you would like to read a great book on this topic, I would suggest Feel the Fear and Do It Anyway, by Susan Jeffers, Ph.D. Although this paperback is a quick read, it is a powerful tool to living life to the fullest.

Fear can be either real or imagined. The mind doesn't differentiate. Eighty percent of what we worry about never happens, so isn't it more realistic to be positive than negative! Why be miserable when we can be happy? We create our own reality. Dr. Jeffers discusses different levels of fear and ways of overcoming them. One of her suggestions is to "just get out and do it!" ACTION CONQUERS FEAR!

THE POWER OF NEGATIVITY

Jack Canfield, one of the authors of the "Chicken Soup Series," uses this demonstration to demonstrate the power of positive versus negative thinking. I have used this same experiment in the classroom to demonstrate the negative effect of items such as sugar, caffeine, and salt on the body.

NEGATIVITY DEMONSTRATIONS

POWER OF WORDS

Have a person stand up and make a fist and extend either arm out to the side. Tell him to resist with as much strength as he can as you attempt to push his arm down with your outstretched hand. Then have him put the arm down, close his eyes, and repeat ten times the negative statement: "I am a weak and unworthy person." Have him really say this expression with emotion, then have him open his eyes, extend his arm out, and, with very little effort, you can bring the arm down. All of his strength has left him. Many will want to repeat the experiment, and the result is always the same. Then have the person close his eyes and repeat ten times the positive statement: "I am a strong and worthy person." Again, he should say these words with feeling. Have him extend his arm and resist your pressure. You will not be able to lower his arm. Positive words mean a strong arm and negative words mean a weak arm. Try it!

FOOD SENSITIVITIES

If you want to test the sensitivity of food items, take six items like coffee, sugar, peanuts, tobacco, salt, and chocolate and put these separately in six envelopes. In the seventh envelope, place nothing. Seal the envelopes and have the individual put one envelope in one hand and place the hand on the side of their leg. They extend the other hand, and you try to pull down on the arm the same as you did in the negativity experiment. Do this with all seven envelopes. You will not be able to push the arm down with the envelope having nothing and probably two or three others, but there may be three or four envelopes in which the arm will offer little resistance. These are the foods to avoid as your body is sensitive to them, and they lower your resistance.

Victor Frankl, who lost his family and loved ones in the German concentration camps during WW II, states in, Man's Search for Meaning that everything can be taken away from a man but one thing: the mind, which enables one to choose one's attitude, regardless of the circumstances.

BOTTOM LINE:

While we can't control the world, we can control our reactions to it.
You have a choice: "Am I going to be miserable or happy? The choice is up to me!"

We need to avoid "PSYCHOSCLEROSIS!" (Hardening of the attitude). My good friend, Murray Banks, who is a motivational speaker and world class athlete, says: "We either choose to make ourselves cynical and tired or we choose to make ourselves positive and enthusiastic. The amount of energy expended is the same ... the trick is in what we choose."

COPING WITH STRESS

POSITIVE	NEGATIVE
1. EXERCISE	1. OVER/UNDER EATING
2. ATTITUDE	2. SEDENTARY
3. PROPER NUTRITION	3. DRUGS
4. ADEQUATE SLEEP	4. SMOKING
5. SPIRITUALITY	5. EXCESS ALCOHOL
6. RELAXATION	6. OVER SPENDING

**DO YOU NEED
AN ATTITUDE
ADJUSTMENT?**

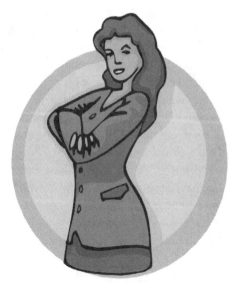

STRESS REACTIVITY

The following are some of the body's reactions to stress:

- Increased heart rate
- Muscle tension
- Rapid, shallow breathing
- Hyperventilation
- Increased blood pressure
- Widening of the pupils of the eyes
- Increased stomach acid
- Opening of the arteries to the heart
- Increased perspiration
- Decrease in the effectiveness of the immune system
- Constriction of the blood vessels in the fingers and toes, leading to being "white as a ghost."

STRESS ILLNESSES

If the stress on the body continues, the above reactions will eventually translate into one or more of the following illnesses:

- High blood pressure
- Cardiovascular (heart) disease
- Migraine headaches
- Cancer
- Asthma
- Rheumatoid arthritis
- Backache
- Stroke
- Ulcers
- Tension headaches
- Allergies
- Hay fever
- Diabetes
- AND ON, AND ON, AND ON…

QUESTION: Would you like a pill that could cure most of these illnesses and many, many more? How much would you pay for it?

ANSWER: EXERCISE IS MORE EFFECTIVE THAN ANY PILL WE HAVE, AND IT IS FREE!

In addition to the above, there are other effects of stress. Generally, poor management of stress is also indicative of poor nutrition, lack of exercise, dependence on the medical system, and reliance on alcohol, tobacco, and other addictive substances.

BOTTOM LINE: THIS LIFESTYLE GUARANTEES TO PRODUCE DISEASE AND PREMATURE DEATH!

When the body encounters a perceived stressor (remember to the body, perception is reality, thus the stressor doesn't have to be real), the nerves send a message to the brain. The brain responds in two ways: one, the brain activates the adrenaline and non-adrenaline hormones (described later in the "fight or flight" syndrome) and two, the pituitary gland is activated. This gland releases a host of chemicals to various organs of the body.

STAGES OF STRESS ACTIVATION

There are three stages of stress activation:

A. Different cycles of electrical activity occur in the brain.

B. The "fight or flight" response is initiated.

C. The general adaptation syndrome kicks in.

The brain records various activity waves depending upon the stimulation.

Delta — Deep Sleep — 1/2 to 4 cycles per second

Theta — Shallow Sleep — 4 to 8 cycles per second

Alpha — Optimal — 8 to 13 cycles per second

Beta — Arousal state — 13 to 32 cycles per second

The obvious goal during our waking hours is to maintain the alpha state. This is accomplished by blanking out the stressors, which will create the mental peace conducive to creativity. By doing this, we will regain normal blood pressure and normal cholesterol levels and lower nervous tension and anxiety. There are several techniques to accomplish this goal, such as affirmations, meditation, progressive relaxation, and exercise. These will be discussed later in this chapter.

Relaxation, Every Day

When the relaxation response is called on, heart rate and blood pressure drop. Breathing rate and oxygen consumption decline because of the profound decrease in the need for energy. Brain waves shift from an alert beta-rhythm to a relaxed alpha-rhythm ... Blood flow to the muscles decreases, and instead, blood is sent to the brain and skin, producing a feeling of warmth and rested alertness. The body reduces the output of adrenaline and cortisol which inhibit the immune system. Relaxation increases the production of interferon, a molecule that boosts the function of natural killer cells and other types of immune cells. Stress is one of many factors that may tip the balance toward illness. Relaxation helps the body heal itself. (Borysenko)

Take Short Naps

Walk, stretch or climb stairs during your break to renew energy and relieve stress. Restore balance with relaxation, meditation and daydreaming

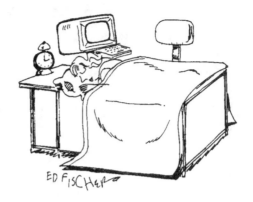

(Reprinted with permission from Dr. Jeff Haebig, Wellness Quest©)

If you only have 2 minutes to relax:

1. Listen to a tape if possible. It can be soothing music or a relaxation tape.
2. Think about what has been bothering you, and then let it be lifted up and taken away.
3. This is your time. There is nothing you need to do now.
4. Picture a place where you would like to be …
5. Close your eyes.
6. Take a deep breath, hold it and let it out.
7. Relax your muscles.
8. Picture yourself in this relaxing place …

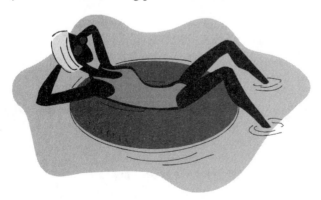

Carolyn Greenlaw RN, BSN, Health Age Resources, Inc. Rockford, Il

"FIGHT OR FLIGHT" SYNDROME:

The good news is that this syndrome was inborn into all of us millions of years ago. It served our ancestors well as they needed a boost of adrenaline before fighting, running, and jumping to avoid being eaten (ugh). The bad news is that we no longer need to resort to those activities, and frequent activation of this response without suitable behavior outlets (i.e. exercise) can lead to the illnesses listed previously. Therefore, we must learn to manage the "fight or flight" syndrome before it manages us.

This syndrome was first documented by the father of stress research, Hans Selye. For those who have had the fortune or misfortune (depending on how you view it) of being involved in wartime activities, this response serves us well. I spent two years in Vietnam, and I had several occasions where this response came into play. I'm thankful it did!

GENERAL ADAPTATION SYNDROME:

There are three stages to this syndrome:

- Alarm Reaction

- Resistance

- Exhaustion

> *"I've known a lot of trouble in life, most of which never happened."*
> — Mark Twain

In the first stage, your body undergoes the biochemical reactions previously described as part of the nonspecific response, and your overall resistance is lowered. In the second stage, resistance increases due to the body's alarm reaction. If this continues over a long period, it eventually leads to the third stage in which your body's energy is depleted, and if that continues, you're in big trouble. Your adaptation energy is finite or limited. Like our bank accounts, some have more in their stress account than others, but eventually stress will deplete your body of the resources it needs to defend itself.

SATCHEL PAIGE'S RULES FOR LIVING RIGHT

1. Avoid fried foods which "angry up" the blood.
2. If your stomach disputes you, lie down and pacify it with cooling thoughts.
3. Keep the juices flowing by jangling around gently as you move.
4. Go very lightly on the vices such as carrying on in society – the social ramble ain't restful.
5. Avoid running at all times.
6. Don't look back, somethin' might be gaining on you.
7. Sometimes I sits and thinks, and sometimes I just sits.

Satchel Paige, 1906-1982. NOTE: Satchel Paige was a black baseball pitcher who, because of discrimination, wasn't able to pitch in the major leagues until he was in his 60's. As you can see, he had his own ideas for stress management.

---

12 PRINCIPLES FOR STRESS MANAGEMENT

Now that we've seen the bad side of stress, let's look at how you can take responsibility for your life and avoid the stress pitfalls by managing the stress before it manages you.

1. Take stock of your own power. Remember Victor Frankl who proved that everything can be taken away from you except your mind. Each of us is unique, and as Dr. George Sheehan used to say, "we're an experiment of one." We all have the resources within ourselves to take control. Distress is NOT what others do to you, but what you do to yourself. Interpret the stressors in a positive way.

2. Make up guidelines that you can live with. Look at the stress management techniques in the next section and decide what fits you.

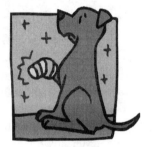

3. Take it easy. Remember the 80/20 Rule. Eighty percent of what we worry about never happens, and if it does, use the FIDO principle. Do what you can about the situation and forget it – FIDO (forget it, drive on).

4. Design working, living, and commuting environments that are quiet and comfortable. The average person spends over an hour a day in his/her vehicle. This is the perfect time to practice stress management techniques.

5. Have a goal bigger than life. This translates into having a purpose. My goal in life is to "make a difference," and I hope to accomplish that objective through this book and programs like "Dump Your Plump™" and Wellness Cruises.

6. Give hugs and pats on the back. Remember, what goes out comes back 10 times.

7. Be pro-active. Prepare ahead of time. Don't make decisions when you're stressed. If you have to make a decision on the spur of the moment, try and respond intellectually to the situation and not react emotionally. There is a difference.

8. Be gently assertive. Look out for your best interests, and let people know your feelings. Don't assume that people can read your mind.

9. For those situations that seem to have no other solution, consider changing the stressful aspects of your life, i.e. job, social group, etc. This may not be easy, but in the long run it could make all the difference.

10. Seek spiritual assistance. For most people this means seeking help from the religion of your choice. There will be more on this principle in the next chapter.

11. Change your perception of the stress-inducing event. The driver who cuts you off in traffic is not trying to run you off the road but a friend who is responding to an emergency. Getting stopped at a railroad crossing or a traffic jam gives you an opportunity to finish reading the newspaper.

12. Understand and deal with your anger. Murray Banks likes to use the Richter Scale in rating your anger level. On a scale of 1-10 is the event that occurred to you a 1 (no effect) or a 10 (deadly) or somewhere in between? What is the rating you assign to the person cutting in front of you in the supermarket line? Is it a 2 or an 8? Will it effect your life two weeks from now, one year from now? How about the loss of your spouse through death or divorce? Is this a 2 or an 8? Decide what's a 10 for you.

STRESS INTERVENTION TECHNIQUES

I will list a dozen or so stress relieving techniques. Pick the ones that fit your personality.

1. Maintain a stress diary. Record as much as you can about the incidents that upset you. Record your emotions, the trigger events, your responses and what you learned from the situation. Just writing the encounter down will relieve some of the stress.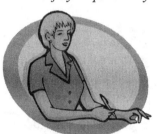

2. Practice selective awareness. As explained in principle 11 above, choose what you want to concentrate on. When you're exercising concentrate on the good you're doing your body and not the difficulty of the activity. One of the best things to remember when you are in a stressful situation is the "Serenity Prayer."

> *"Lord, give me the courage to change the things I can, the serenity to accept the things that I can't, and the wisdom to know the difference."* — Rheinhold Neibuhr

3. Practice time management. This is an important principle and there are many good books on the subject. One of the first and still the best books on this subject is,

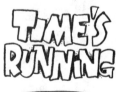

Seven Habits of Highly Effective People by Steven Covey. The seven habits, such as creating a win/win situation and being proactive are discussed. The habit I like is, "Habit 3. Put First things First." (Covey)

For this he draws up a time management matrix with how we should be spending the majority of our time in Category II (important - not urgent.) You'll have to read the book to see why you don't want to spend the majority of your time in Category I (important - urgent.) I'll give you a hint - the person in Category I is always putting out fires.

COVEY'S TIME MANAGEMENT CHART

	URGENT	NOT URGENT
IMPORTANT	I	II
NOT IMPORTANT	III	IV

4. Practice good nutrition. Do you eat foods for fuel or to make your mouth smile? Foods such as caffeine, sugar, salt, alcohol, and fat are empty calories and are setting you up for problems down the road. Fruits and vegetables provide the basis for an immune-boosting diet. Foods are no longer fats, proteins and carbohydrates, but bio-chemically active substances that can be of value in fighting disease.

The natural form of soluble fiber known as psyllium helps with diarrhea and constipation. Vitamin B6 is essential for proper brain and nerve function. Vitamin C is helpful in fighting off colds, healing cuts, and decreasing seasonal allergies, and Vitamin E is credited with reducing heart disease risk and preventing heart attacks. You must eat right knowing the benefits of vitamin and mineral substances to assist your body with all the stresses of job, family, and disease. Remember you are what you eat!

5. Avoid tobacco, alcohol, and other addictive substances. 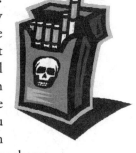 Avoiding cigarettes should go without saying. I feel very strongly that cigarettes should be illegal. Cigarettes claimed my dad's life at 48 years of age. I was only 8 years old, a fact I will never forget which is why I campaign hard for smoking restrictions. I call cigarettes, "cancerettes." They are designed with one purpose in mind and that is to kill you. If you don't believe me, look at the black, charred lung of a smoker. Remember, each cigarette you put in your mouth takes 15 minutes off your life. The same can be said for the other addictive substances. Please stay away from them.

6. Practice effective learning. We are never too old to stop learning. According to the experts, knowledge keeps doubling every 5-10 years. If we stop learning the new methods and equipment, we're setting ourselves up for stress down the road. Not having a working knowledge of the computer today is similar to the person in the 1960's who could not read or write.

7. Try different mental activities to relax yourself.

a. Meditation: This is a practice that goes way back to the ancient Eastern and Western civilizations. You make a concentrated effort to focus on a physical experience, sound, or thought to bring peace of mind and aid in healing. Meditation reduces your body's response to stress and can lead to improved symptoms of stress related conditions. Doctors have prescribed meditation as a way to lower blood pressure, ease asthma and generally relax.

b. Prayer: This is a very effective form of meditation. Prayer will be covered in greater detail in the next chapter. For now, we will simply say that prayer makes a difference!

c. Relaxation Response: The person credited with the secular Relaxation Response is Dr. Herbert Benson of the Harvard Medical School. Dr. Benson was one of the first medical doctors to study the health benefits of prayer and meditation. Benson showed that when the subjects trained their mind to focus on a word, sound, prayer, phrase, or an activity such as jogging, swimming, or even knitting that healthful bodily changes occurred-lower blood pressure, and slower heart rate. He found that the results were the same whether the person used words with secular meaning, i.e., one, ocean, love, peace, calm, and relax or religious focus words like "Jesus" or "God" or prayers such as the first line of the Lords Prayer: "Our Father, who art in heaven." (Benson)

RELAXATION RESPONSE *by Herbert Benson*

1. QUIET ENVIRONMENT:
For 10-20 minutes.

2. OBJECT TO CONCENTRATE ON:
Can be a word, sound, phrase, or feeling. Repeat object constantly, silently, and with eyes closed.

3. PASSIVE ATTITUDE:
Let it happen. If distracting thoughts occur, do not worry. Just return to the object.

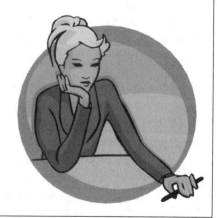

4. COMFORTABLE POSITION:
One that you can stay in at least 20 minutes (usually sitting.)

Practice Twice a Day if Possible

---

d. Visualization: This is a powerful tool for improving physical or mental performance and relieving stress. It has many applications. One of the best examples of the power of visualization occurred during the Vietnam War. An Air Force pilot was captured by the North Vietnamese and imprisoned for five years. Prior to his capture, he was an avid golfer but a very poor one, struggling to break 100 strokes for 18 holes. When he was released from captivity, the first thing he did when he reached Hawaii was to play a round of golf with his friends, and he proceeded to shoot par golf or 72. His friends couldn't believe it so they had him play another round the next day and he repeated the low score. They asked him what had happened. Before he was captured, he was a duffer, and after five years in a 5' by 5' cell, he had become a very proficient golfer. His answer was that every day for five years he had played a round of golf in his head. It took him four hours to complete the round. He visualized the sand traps, putting, driving, and all the nuances of golf. This is a terrific example showing that the mind can't distinguish between the real and the imaginary. Professional athletes in all sports, tennis, bowling, basketball, baseball, football, etc. visualize themselves as being successful. The important thing is to visualize successful shots and plays. The more vivid you can make the visualizations, the better.

I used this concept with my students. For example, during bowling class, as they took their stance, they would visualize themselves making the correct approach and releasing the ball for a successful roll of the ball to a strike.

Another form of visualization is daydreams. When your body yearns for a break and your mind craves tranquility, let the power of your imagination transport you to peaceful places in your mind. Perhaps a sun swept mountaintop, a cozy cabin retreat, an invigorating sail, a bubbling hot spring. The possibilities are endless. Visit these places for 5-10 minutes.

e. Journaling: Journaling is a powerful tool for keeping track of the ups and downs in your search for a healthy balance. Writing about yourself is a form of "talking to yourself" without being heard. As you progress through the process, you will discover new insights about yourself that will teach you lessons you need to know.

f. Music: Music is a very popular choice to alleviate stress, insomnia, and depression. Music has proven to reverse stress related conditions and improve concentration and memory. If you want assistance in the selection of appropriate music, look for a registered music therapist (RMT). In my estimation, it is better to listen to Beethoven than the Beach Boys. According to a noted psychiatrist, "30 minutes of Beethoven equals 10 mg of Valium."

TOP 10 MYTHS ABOUT MEDITATION

MYTH: You need to sit in a lotus position.
FACT: You can meditate in any position, i.e. sitting, walking, standing or lying down.

MYTH: You need absolute quiet.
FACT: You can meditate anywhere. If you're paying attention to your meditation you will block out the background noise. If you are temporarily distracted by "clutter" simply redirect your attention back to your thoughts. Losing focus is not a cause to blame yourself.

MYTH: You need to mediate by using religious thoughts or words.
FACT: Spiritual meditation is one choice you have. However, you can meditate by using thoughts of beautiful scenery such as the serenity of "Red Rock Crossing" in Arizona, an enjoyable physical activity or using words like "peace" or "love."

MYTH: You need to study first.
FACT: Knowledge is not essential. Whatever is important to you will provide a moving experience. Someone once said that when it comes to meditation you can't do it wrong.

MYTH: Meditation is for passive people.
FACT: Meditating doesn't mean that you let people walk all over you. Instead it helps you make intelligent, deliberate decisions. By meditating first before acting, you tend to make better decisions. I recall in one of my college education classes, the point was made that teachers must learn to "act and not react."

MYTH: You'll become unemotional or detached.
FACT: Meditation doesn't mean that you eliminate the ups and downs of life, but rather it helps smooth out he emotional rollercoaster ride that tend to get into.

MYTH: Meditation means you can't have an active life:
FACT: You can work meditation into your daily life , no matter how busy you may be. You can have a purposeful walk, a meditative weight training session or a mindful meditation while you're doing household chores.

MYTH: Meditation is too hard to learn.
FACT: Anything worthwhile takes time to learn, but is ultimately worth it. Learning to play tennis, golf or play the piano takes perseverance, but half the enjoyment is in the journey.

MYTH: Meditation is a selfish activity.

FACT: I once had an older college student who said that she set aside 30 minutes every morning to go for a walk. By doing this, she said, it makes me a better mother, wife and a healthier person. It is essential that we set aside time to nurture our bodies.

MYTH: Meditation is a religion.

FACT: This is an absolute falsehood. That's like saying that when you're stressed, deep breathing shouldn't be done because it means that you're practicing an Eastern religion. I know of school systems that forbid their teachers from the teaching the technique of deep breathing because of this connotation. What a shame! Taking a deep breath when you're stressed is a technique that should be taught to every student.

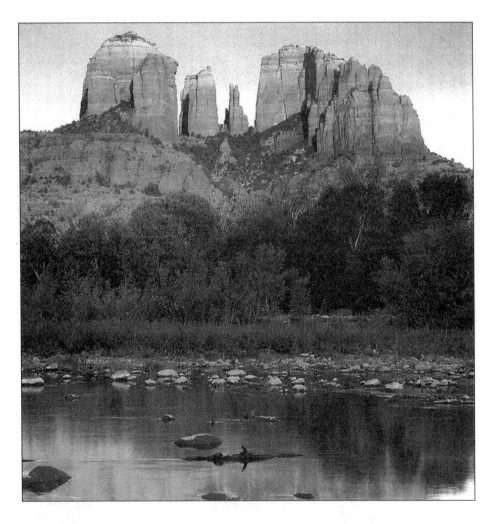

My favorite meditation spot — Red Rock Crossing

g. **Affirmations:** These are my favorite tool for reducing stress. Affirmations are self-talk in its highest form. Remember the power of self talk in the arm experiment? Affirmations are the easiest and cheapest stress reduction tools you can use. An affirmation is a POSITIVE statement that something is already happening. It's not happening tomorrow or in the future but right now. The rules for affirmations are simple. The first rule is, always state your affirmation in the present. For example, "I now weigh 150 lbs.," not, "I will weigh 150 lbs." The second rule is, always state it in the positive, rather than the negative. "I will not miss a day of exercise," might be, "I look forward to and enjoy exercising every day."

HERE ARE A FEW EXAMPLES OF AFFIRMATIONS:

- "I can feel the energy going through my body."
- "I can see and feel my muscles getting stronger."
- "My world is filled with peace and happiness."
- "I am handling all of my fears."

RULES FOR MAKING AFFIRMATIONS

"I am exercising every day and love it."

- Personal   "I"
- Positive   "am"
- Present tense   "exercising"
- Specific   "every day"
- Feeling words   "love it"
- Brief   "KISS (Keep It Short and Simple)
- Personal   Not for others

DON'S FAVORITE AFFIRMATIONS

Affirmation for rising in the morning.

AS MY EYES OPEN TO THE LIGHT, I SAY TO MYSELF,

"What a Wonderful World!"

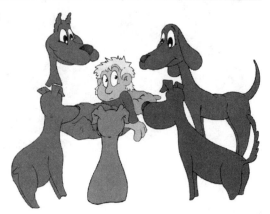

AS I'M SHAVING, I REPEAT THIS AFFIRMATION:

"This is the beginning of a new day. God has given me this day to use as I will. What I do today is important because I'm exchanging a day of my life for it. When tomorrow comes, today will be gone forever, leaving in its place that which I have traded for. I want it to be gain, not loss, good not evil, so that I will not regret the price that I paid for it."
— *ANONYMOUS*

WHEN I'M EXERCISING I SAY,

"I am creating a strong, healthy body. I can feel the energy going through my body."

THROUGHOUT THE DAY I SAY,

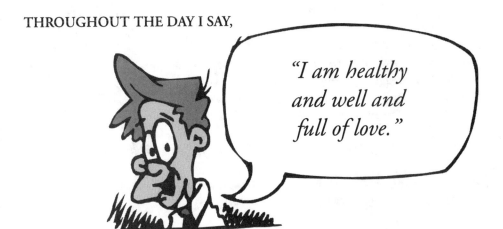

"I am healthy and well and full of love."

RULES FOR USING AFFIRMATIONS

Put 5-10 affirmations on 3x5 cards. Place them in conspicuous places throughout your home so that you see them when...

- You get out of bed
- You're dressing,
- You're using the bathroom
- You're opening the refrigerator
- etc.

Put the cards in your pocket and several times a day pull them out and read them. If you have supportive friends, share your affirmations with them and ask them to support you.

www.knowitbyheart.com
This company produces affirmations on shirts, cards, videos, and books.

225

8. Physical Activities To Relax Yourself: The following are just a few ideas that you might want to check out.

a. Massage uses various techniques to manipulate body tissue for therapeutic purposes. It works by increasing circulation, thereby relieving tension and pain, allowing toxins in the body to dissipate. There are more than 100 massage methods, so if one form doesn't produce results, try another.

b. Give yourself a massage with "The Stick."

THE STICK

The "Stick" is an award-winning, non-motorized instrument for the management of over-used, over-worked muscle. It easily molds to various body types and can be used on all major muscle groups - may be used through clothing or directly on the skin. The Stick provides instant myofascial release, meaning relaxed, healthy muscle fibers encourage good circulation. Adequate blood supply allows muscle to feel better, work harder, last longer, and recover faster. It can be used by yourself or with another person.

For information on purchasing The Stick call Rainbow Wellness at 269-925-3524 or go to www.dumpyourplump.com

---

c. Hot tubs and saunas are favorites of mine. They increase circulation and thus speed healing. Hydrotherapy is the easiest therapy to master for home use. I have considerable osteoarthritis, and the warm water does wonders for relieving the muscle pain.

d. Tai Chi, Qigong, Yoga and Pilates are all disciplines that have become accepted in the American Wellness field. They are designed to promote flexibility, breathing and body alignment. For a more detailed description, refer to the chapter on Complementary and Alternative Medicine (CAM).

e. Progressive Relaxation: This is a technique of scanning your body in search of accumulated tension. This is done by starting at the top or bottom of the body and gradually progressing upward or downward, tightening and relaxing the different muscle groupings.   A comforting relaxation will spread through your body, and once you have felt it, you will be able to recall that relaxed feeling when you start to feel your body becoming tense.

f. Relaxation Breathing: (4-7-8) Use this technique when you feel tension building up. First, place the tip of your tongue just behind the upper front teeth and keep it there throughout the whole exercise.

1) Inhale deeply and quietly through your nose to a silent count of 4 (w/mouth closed).

2) Hold the breath for a count of 7.

3) Exhale through your mouth to a count of 8, making a whoosh sound.

* This is one breath. Now repeat the entire cycle three or more times

9. Humor: The power of humor in the treatment of serious illness, including stress, is well documented. Norman Cousins in Anatomy of an Illness, laid the ground work for the place of humor in the treatment of an illness. He watched "Marx Brothers" movies and "I Love Lucy" reruns to give himself belly laughs. You may not need a cure for a physical illness but a cure for the 'blahs'. Kids laugh at least 400 times a day, whereas adults laugh 15 or less times a day.

When was the last time you had a good belly laugh?

My good friend, Dr. Jeff Haebig, has developed several programs: "Quick Quest," Health Care-toon Calendars, and the "Brain/Body Boogie." The "Quick Quest" program captures people's fancy as wellness challenges are completed and celebrated. The desktop, undated Health Care-toon Calendar keeps the wellness messages in front of people on a daily basis. Several of the cartoons in this book come from Jeff's programs. If you desire an energetic, dynamic speaker, Jeff will fill the bill. He conducts interactive workshops for students, families, corporations, and communities. He will lead the audience in activities such as the "Wellness Shuffle" or the "Brain/Body Boogie." For more information on Dr. Haebig's award winning programs, visit his web site at: www.wellnessquest.com.

> **PROVERB 17:22**
>
> "A cheerful heart is good medicine, but a broken spirit saps a person's strength."

BENEFITS OF HUMOR

- **PHYSICAL:** HUMORAEROBICS - reaches every body organ.
- **SOCIAL:** SOCIAL LUBRICANT - breaks down barriers.
- **PSYCHOLOGICAL:** INSTANT VACATION.
- **SPIRITUAL:** COMIC AND COSMIC VIEW OF LIFE.

HUMOR AS A HEALER:

Humor Prescription:

WHO: Anyone

WHAT: Find a form of humor that gives you a good belly laugh.

WHEN: Whenever possible.

WHERE: Everywhere.

WHY: Life should be enjoyed.

HOW: Look for humor. It's all around you!

Wouldn't it be nice to receive this prescription?

Larry Ulery, MA, CHES, Andrews University, Berrien Springs, MI

10. Social Support: This topic has been discussed throughout this book. It doesn't matter whether it's exercising, losing weight, stopping an addictive behavior, or dealing with stress, the help of a friend makes all the difference. That is why I encouraged you at the beginning of the book to draw up a buddy contract. A buddy should be someone that will encourage you and make you feel wonderful about yourself. When you are changing habits, you don't want to be around negative people. The type of friends you want are not energy takers, but givers. They are a joy to be around. If you can't find these kind of friends, then find a support group. There are many support groups out there, and they are definitely worth taking the time to find.

11. Exercise, exercise, exercise: A vital step in the regulation of stress is a REGULAR exercise program. In this day and age, where stress is at an all-time high, our bodies kick out stress hormones, which if not used for their intended purpose (fight or flight), then circulate through the body, causing damage to various organs, including the immune system.

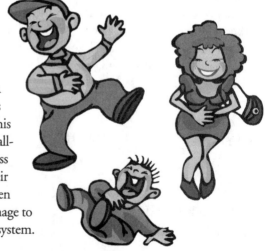

Physical activity is considered the best way to keep the physiological systems of the body in balance. The important thing is that the exercise benefit can be plugged in at any level on the stress model. However, the earlier it is used, the better. Exercise may stress the body, but it de-stresses the mind. The Romans had it right when they said, "Mens sana in corpore sano (A sound mind in a sound body)." One supports the other.

§, Exercise When Stressed

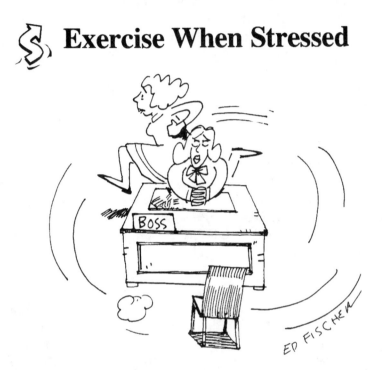

(Reprinted with permission from Dr. Jeff Haebig, Wellness Quest©)

12. Relaxation tapes for surgery: I discovered these tapes several years ago when I was having hip surgery. There is a series of six tapes. I listened to the Hemi-Sync tapes for several days preceding the surgery, during the pre-operation procedures, during surgery, in the recovery room, and during recuperation. I recall that when I was in the pre-op area and they first took my blood pressure it was 190/140 as I was very tense about the upcoming operation. I listened to the tapes for 60 minutes, and the last thing I remember before being put to sleep was that the blood pressure, was 90/60. The doctors and nurses were amazed at the small loss of blood during surgery, as I didn't even use one unit of blood (my circulation system had been slowed down), the lessened pain, and the rapidity of healing that took place. I have used these tapes in several operations since, my wife has used them in her operations, and we have loaned them out to friends. In every situation, they have reduced the pain and recovery process. Numerous studies have documented that tapes such as these speed up tremendously the healing process. It's amazing that they are not used more.

HEMI-SYNC

The Monroe Institute is a pioneer in its work with audio sound patterns that have become known as "Hemi-Sync." They have discovered how to produce an electrical signal that requires both hemispheres of the brain to be working together. Their tapes can be used for weight loss, memory improvement, relaxation, medical rehabilitation, surgery, sleeping, and the grieving process.

For information on these tapes call toll free: 1-866-881-3440
or go to www.monroeinstitute.org.

13. Get A Pet: The late Charles Schulz, creator of "Peanuts" had a quote, "Happiness is a warm puppy." Will Rogers used to say that "the outside of a horse was good for the inside of man." My wife and I have found great pleasure with our four dachshunds, "Benno," "Lynkey," "Kristl," and now "Heidi," but we've found similar pleasure with our cat, "Boots." Studies have repeatedly shown that people with pets live longer and have a better quality of life. GET A PET!

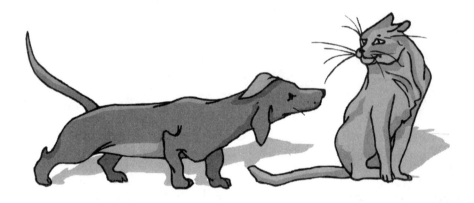

14. Go Outside: Develop a deep connection to nature. Experience ways (hiking, canoeing, rafting, mountain climbing) to rejuvenate your physical, psychological, and spiritual well-being. Even if it's just looking at an aquarium for 30 minutes, visiting a garden, or viewing landscape photography, it gives you a lift.

15. Go Fishing: "If people concentrated on the really important things in life, there'd be a shortage of fishing poles."

Bruce Larson

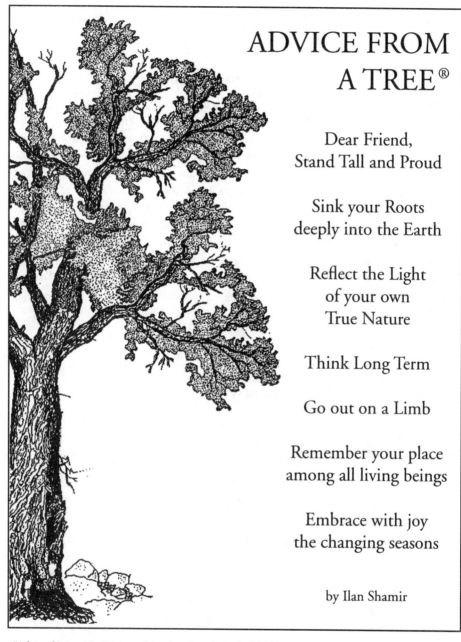

ADVICE FROM
A TREE ®

Dear Friend,
Stand Tall and Proud

Sink your Roots
deeply into the Earth

Reflect the Light
of your own
True Nature

Think Long Term

Go out on a Limb

Remember your place
among all living beings

Embrace with joy
the changing seasons

by Ilan Shamir

"Advice from a Tree" is copyrighted and trademarked by Your True Nature. Used with permission.

Ilan Shamir, author of "Advice from a Tree," made his niche in the business world when he created the slogan, "7-Up, the UnCola." He has since turned his creative talents into creating the "Advice from a Tree" and "A Thousand Things Went Right Today" programs. 910-282-1620 (www.yourtruenature.com)

"I'd Pick More Daisies"

If I had my life to live over, I'd try to make more mistakes next time. I would relax, I would limber up, I would be sillier than I have been this trip. I know of very few things I would take seriously. I would be crazier, I would be less nervous, I would take more chances, I would take more trips. I would climb more mountains, swim more rivers, watch more sunsets. I would eat more ice cream and few beans. I would have more actual troubles and fewer imaginary ones. You see, I'm one of those people who have lived their lives sensibly and sanely, hour after hour, day after day. Oh, I've had my moments and if I had to do it over again, I'd have more of them. In fact, I'd try to do nothing else, just moments, one after another, instead of living so many years ahead of each day. I've been one of those people who never go anywhere without a thermometer, a hot water bottle, a gargle, a raincoat and a parachute. If I had to do it over, I'd start barefoot earlier in the spring and stay that way until late in the fall. I'd play more hookey, I wouldn't get such good grades except by accident. I'd ride on more merry-go-rounds. I'd pick more daisies. — Anonymous

The Final Analysis

People are often unreasonable, illogical, and self centered...
FORGIVE THEM ANYWAY.

If you are kind, people may accuse you of selfish ulterior motives...
BE KIND ANYWAY.

If you are successful, you will win some friends and some enemies...
SUCCEED ANYWAY.

If you are honest and frank, people may cheat you...
BE HONEST AND FRANK ANYWAY.

What you spend years building, someone could destroy overnight...
BUILD ANYWAY.

If you find serenity and happiness, they may be jealous...
BE HAPPY ANYWAY.

The good you do today, people will often forget tomorrow...
DO GOOD ANYWAY.

Give the world the best you have and it may never be enough...
GIVE THE WORLD THE BEST YOU'VE GOT ANYWAY.

You see, in the final analysis, it is between you and God...
IT WAS NEVER BETWEEN YOU AND THEM ANYWAY.

— Mother Teresa

CHAPTER TWELVE:
SPIRITUALITY:
THE FORGOTTEN FACTOR
OF WELLNESS

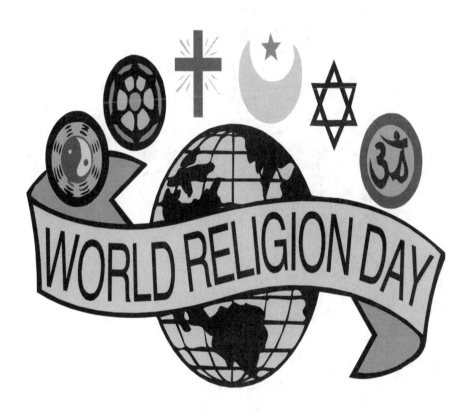

"Never forget, Americans, that yours is a spiritual country. Yes, I know you're a practical people. Like others, I've marveled at your factories, your skyscrapers, and your arsenals. But, underlying everything else is the fact that America began as a God-loving, God-fearing, God-worshipping, people."

General Romulo, General of the Philippines

THE SECOND 10 COMMANDMENTS

by Stephen Yarnell, M.D.

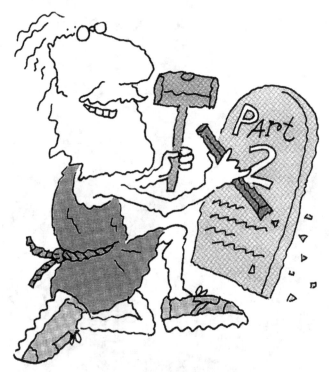

THOU SHALT:

Exercise Thy Body

Exercise Thy Mind

Exercise Thy Spirit

Exercise Thy Willpower

Have a Happy Heart

Eat, Drink & Be Merry – Sensibly

Play

Give up Guilt, Regret and Depression

Fear Not the Future

Live Now

SPIRITUALITY VS. RELIGION

This chapter will not discuss specific religions, but rather the basic core values that make up spiritual health. Spirituality is neither a religion nor the practice of a religion. Spirituality is a belief that we are connected to, and dependent upon, something outside of ourselves, whether that something is nature, each other, or the unknown. Religion is a specific belief system that defines and explains that connection.

It is my observation that spirituality is a uniting factor, whereas religions sometimes tend to divide. Spiritual health is not determined by the rituals of organized religion but rather by your answers to the questions of, Who am I? Where did I come from? What are my basic values? Where do I fit into the big picture? and finally, Where am I going to spend eternity? Human spirituality is not bound by the confines of religious dogma. The issues of relationships, personal values, and the meaning of life go beyond the limitations of culture, religion, and egos.

> *"The existing definition of health should include the spiritual aspect and that health care should be in the hands of those who are fully aware of and sympathetic to the spiritual dimension."*
>
> — World Health Organization

"No matter how diverse we are, there is a common bond in the spirit of God that can bring us together." Those sentiments were echoed by Catholic Cardinal Adam Maida at a public worship of local bishops, imans, rabbis, and priests, celebrating the 300th birthday of Detroit, Michigan. At the conclusion of the celebration, Trilochem Singh, a Sikh said, "We are children of the same God. Whether we go to a church, a synagogue, a mosque or a temple, we pray for the same things."

Throughout the ages, the scriptures of all religions have proclaimed that humanity is one great family. This sameness is reflected in the principles of religious thought that are expressed very similarly in every religion. The principles of: "Love Thy Neighbor," "Honor Thy Father and Mother," "Speak Truth," "Man does not live by bread alone," and "It is more blessed to give than to receive," are just a few philosophies shared by all of the religions.

THE POWER OF PRAYER

"Don't pray when it rains, if you don't pray when the sun shines."
Satchel Paige (1906-1982)

"Pray as if everything depended upon God and work as if everything depended upon man."
Cardinal Francis Spellman (1989-1987)

"Prayer indeed is good, but while calling in the gods a man should himself lend a hand."
Hippocrates (460-377 BC)

"The time to pray is not when we are in a tight spot, but just as soon as we get out of it."
Josh Billings (1818-1885)

"Give us this day our daily bread," is probably the most perfectly constructed and useful sentence ever set down in the English language.
P.J. Wingate

"Prayer is when you talk to God; meditation is when you LISTEN to God."
Author Unknown

"You should pray for a sound mind in a sound body."
Juvenal (55-127 AD)

"When we pray to God, we must be seeking nothing — nothing."
Sir Francis of Assisi

"When at night you cannot sleep, talk to the Shepherd and stop counting sheep."   Author Unknown

"Many people pray as if God were a big aspirin pill, they come only when they hurt."   Oswald Chambers

"The Lord's Prayer may be committed to memory quickly, but it is slowly learned by heart."   Frederich Denison Maurice

"Prayer connects me to that which is divine in the world. I believe that a spark of divinity resides in each of us, and so prayer not only connects me with God, whom I recognize as the source of all things, it connects me with my fellow travelers on this road of life."
Karen Rosenstein

THE UNIVERSALITY OF THE GOLDEN RULE

- Do unto others as you would have them do unto you, for this is the law and the prophets. — Christianity

- What is hurtful to yourself, do not do to your fellow man. That is the whole of the Torah and the remainder is but commentary. — Judaism

- Do unto all men as you would wish to have done unto you; and reject for others what you would reject for yourselves. — Islam

- Hurt not others with that which pains yourself. — Buddhism

- Tzu - Kung asked: "Is there one principle upon which one's whole life may proceed?" The Master replied, "Is not Reciprocity such a principle?- what you do not yourself desire, do not put before others. — Confucianism

- This is the sum of all true righteousness - Treat others, as thou wouldst thyself be treated. Do nothing to thy neighbor, which hereafter thou wouldst not have thy neighbor do to thee. — Hinduism

ONENESS: Great Principles Shared by All Religions — Jeffery Moses

The purpose of this chapter is to advance spiritual health. I personally belong to a large Protestant denomination and because of several "wake-up calls" in my life, I have a strong belief in God. However, that may not be your belief. Each person has to answer that question for him/herself. Feel free to translate the examples in this chapter into whatever language and perspective that is meaningful to you.

At the beginning of the book, I defined total wellness as "the physical, mental, emotional, social, and spiritual dimension of a person's life." We have discussed the first four dimensions; now it is time to discuss the spiritual aspect. Many wellness providers place spirituality at the core of wellness. Despite the recognized importance of spiritual wellness, it is fair to say that spiritual well-being has been short changed in the area of health promotion. As a matter of fact, in many wellness programs, it has been ignored.

Don Tubesing, MDiv, PhD, a pioneer in the wellness field, expresses it best when he says, "America has neglected the spiritual dimension of life. Therefore, we don't know as much about the spiritual dimension as we do about the physical side. But the spiritual side is the most important dimension of wellness."

It is relatively easy to assess your blood pressure, cholesterol, and fitness level. It is much more difficult to talk about relationships, values, and life's meaning. However, there now appears to be a yearning to go beyond numbers, especially at the workplace where stress and violence are at an all-time high.

SPIRITUALITY IN THE WORKPLACE

There is a growing faith-at-work movement, seeking to increase the presence of religion in the workplace. A 2003 directory published by Business for Social Responsibility lists more than 1200 Christian groups devoted to work place ministry. This is more than double the number of groups that existed five years ago.

Faith in the Workplace Benefits: *(Source: Business for Social Responsibility)*

- Increasing job satisfaction and employee morale
- Boosting employee loyalty and commitment
- Enhancing productivity
- Increasing ability to recruit and retain employees
- Reducing employee stress
- Reducing employee turnover

Spirituality in the workplace has been mistakenly seen as meaning religion in the workplace. Yet, spirituality in the workplace has nothing to do with any religious affiliation. Aspects of workplace spirituality involve, caring for self and community, ethics, counseling, creativity, productivity, and profit.

There appears to be a nationwide trend toward public expressions of spirituality. Each year there is a National Day of Prayer recognized by Congress. More and more corporations are participating in this event. Ford Motor Company has approved the establishment of an Interfaith Network group designed to encourage diversity in the workplace. On National Prayer Day, May 3, 2001, a service led by Protestants, Catholics, Hindus, Muslims, and Jews was held. The service contained Catholic and Protestant prayers, Hindus singing an ancient Sanskrit hymn, Muslims chanting from the Koran, and a Jewish invocation. No clergy were involved. The service was designed and led by Ford workers exploring the tricky landscape of interfaith relations with their coworkers. Invitations were extended through the company e-mail.

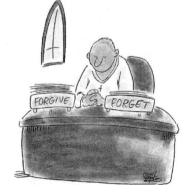

One worker who led the Jewish invocation said: "I'm really impressed that Ford would do this. This is very unusual. At work, most of us have never revealed to each other what our prayers are like. When we come together like this and learn more about each others' faiths, we realize that there's a great deal we can work on together." ("Praise was out loud, at work," Detroit Free Press, May 4, 2001.)

Martin Inglis, head of Ford North American Operations said, "The purpose of the Interfaith Network is not to impose faith on anyone. But faith is a part of who people are and how they feel about themselves. Allowing people to express their faith in a way that is appropriate is great." Another spokesman asked, "How can you ask people to check their hearts at the door when they come to work?"

Is there a place for the Bible in corporate America? People look at religion now as more central to who they are and they come to work with that religious piece of themselves. Zig Ziglar recently did a column on why corporations should encourage this trend. He says that if employees don't follow Biblical principles they will be fired. **THOSE PRINCIPLES ARE:**

- Kill not.

- Steal, gossip, and spread false rumors, not.

- Be kind, tenderhearted and forgiving.

- Give to the poor and encourage the weak.

> **AREN'T THESE THE PRINCIPLES YOU WANT TO ENCOURAGE IN YOUR COMPANY?**

> *Simple Etiquette Rule:*
>
> *Manners guru, Emily Post in her 1922 classic, "Etiquette in Society, in Business, in Politics and at Home," gave the number one rule in etiquette: "Never do anything that is unpleasant to others."*

SPIRITUALITY AND MEDICINE

The medical field is where a big paradigm shift has occurred. Patient demand, coupled with scientific studies correlating faith with good health, is converting a skeptical medical community. Doctors are attending conferences on faith in increasing numbers. In 1996, the Association of American Medical Colleges conducted an extensive study of patients, insurance companies, and the medical community. Cultural, spiritual and end-of-life issues were the dominant themes. In 1995 only a few medical schools taught spirituality. Now some 80 of the 125 U.S. medical schools have required curriculum on the subject.

More doctors are looking at the link between spirituality and healing because their patients already believe in it. Deepak Chopra's series of books on the mind-body connection, Bill Moyer's PBS series and book, <u>Healing and the Mind</u> and Jon Kabat-Zinn's book, <u>Whereas You Go, There You Are</u> are just a few of many publications out there. There are over 800 studies showing that religious faith is related to improved physical and mental heath.

In a 1996 USA Weekend Poll of 1,000 adults, 82% believed that spiritual faith can help people recover from illness, injury, or disease; 56% said their faith has helped them recover from illness, injury or disease; 64% believe doctors should talk to patients about spiritual faith, and yet only 10% say that a doctor has talked to them about their spiritual faith as a factor in physical health. Yet, there are literally hundreds of medical studies documenting the link between faith and health. Their findings show that spiritual people have…

A. **LONGER LIFE.** A nationwide study found a seven-year difference in life expectancy between those who never attend religious services and those who attend more than once a week.

B. **BETTER RECOVERY.** Those patients comforted by their faith had three times the chance of being alive six months after open-heart surgery than patients who found no comfort in religion.

C. **LOWER BLOOD PRESSURE.** A lower blood pressure was found among those who attended church regularly and considered religion important.

D. **BETTER MENTAL HEALTH.** Those attending church had lower rates of depression and anxiety.

> *"Beloved, I wish above all things, that thou mayest prosper and be in health, even as thy soul prospereth."* — 3 John: 2 • King James Version

These studies are just the tip of the iceberg, supporting the contention that both quality and quantity of life is influenced by spirit and religion. But, according to psychiatrist Martin Jones of Howard University College of Medicine, we don't have to wait until all the scientific research is in. "We don't understand the mechanism of many drugs. We know from observing cause and effect that they work. Likewise, we can see the effects of a person's spiritual consciousness on his outcome, so why not use that?"

"Praying affects epinephrine and other stress hormones in the body leading to lower blood pressure, more relaxed heart rate and respiration as well as other benefits."

— Herbert Benson, Harvard University

What are the benefits of being spiritual?

A. BALANCE: Brian Luke Seaward, Ph.D., speaker and author of several books on spirituality, speaks to the importance of finding balance in our lives. He cites an ancient Chinese proverb, "Stand like mountain, move like water." According to Seaward, "Standing like a mountain means to feel strong and secure in the midst of change. To move like water means to go with the flow. In times such as these, where change is ever present, balance is necessary to stay grounded, centered and connected. Time of change brings with it stress, and it is no coincidence that in times of stress, our sights turn toward the heavens for help."

> *Everything on earth has its own time and its own season. There is a time for birth and death, planting and reaping.* — Ecclesiastes 3:1-2

BALANCE?

We are running so fast God, and we don't know to slow down.

We keep our calendars filled.

We carry phones in the car and pagers in the purse.

We constantly check our voice mail, our e-mail and stay connected by fax and Internet.

We are busy and yet not satisfied.

We are moving faster, but we never catch up.

We are stressed, God.

Is this the way you meant us to be?

— Anonymous

B. HEALTH: Health statistics have already been cited, showing that people with spiritual beliefs live longer and have better quality lives. According to Herbert Benson, MD, founder of the Relaxation Response and author of Timeless Healing, the Biology of Belief, "We are wired for God. We have a tremendous healing capacity if we can tap into what I call the 'faith factor." (Benson)

Dale Matthews, MD, in The Faith Factor, cites many studies that show the positive role of faith on well-being, including a stronger immune system, less high blood pressure, faster recoveries from depression and anxiety, shorter hospital stays, better survival rate following surgeries, fewer medications, and better mental health.

C. PURPOSE: Your spiritual life can answer the haunting questions of "Who am I and Why do I exist?," "Where do I go when I die?," and "What is my purpose on earth?" Even the answer to pain and suffering comes from the spiritual realm. Victor Frankl in Man's Search for Meaning found that "Suffering ceases to be suffering once it takes on meaning." He was able to endure the horrors of the concentration camp during the Holocaust with his strong spiritual faith.

D. CONNECTED: Being spiritual connects you with others. As the saying goes, "No man is an island, no man stands alone." We need each other. Your spirituality increases a desire to reach out to others. Relationships with others are enhanced. Your spiritual bond with other people is stronger. Love overflows to others. Love is healing. A survey of 10,000 men found that there was a 50% reduction in the frequency of chest pain of those who perceived that their wives were supportive and loving. Many studies have documented that people with strong social support live longer.

E. SPIRITUALITY: Being spiritual helps you cope with life and stress in a calmer, more peaceful way. You have the belief that "everything works out for the good." For many people, spirituality gives hope when life throws them a curve. Psalm 23 is a promise of peace and calm.

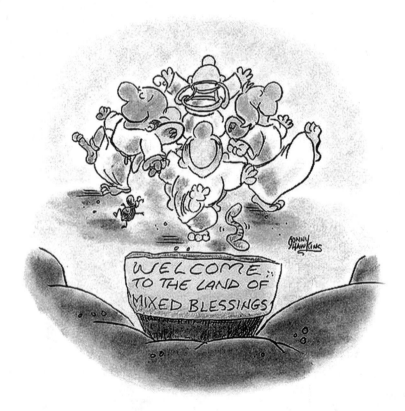

THE GOOD SHEPHERD

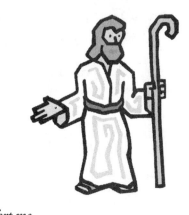

The Lord is my shepherd; I shall not want.

He maketh me to lie down in green pastures:

he leadeth me beside the still waters.

He restoreth my soul: he leadeth me in the

paths of righteousness for his name's sake.

Yea, though I walk through the valley

of the shadow of death, I will fear no evil:

for thou art with me; thy rod and thy staff they comfort me.

Thou preparest a table before me in the presence of mine enemies:

thou anointest my head with oil; my cup runneth over.

Surely goodness and mercy shall follow me all the days of my life:

and I will dwell in the house of the Lord forever.

— (King James version of PSALM 23 - A Psalm of David)

As I mentioned in the stress chapter, we can't control the wind, but we can adjust the sails. Storms will come into everyone's life, but life can be put into perspective when you have a strong spiritual connection.

F. **POWER:** Spirituality gives power to be temperate among all the temptations. All day long you are up against tough choices … donuts on the counter, candy and pop in the vending machine, fast food places on the way home, TV and the Internet that keep you from exercising. How can you make good wellness choices with all of these temptations? Tap into your spiritual power. This may be just the edge you need to make positive choices. Start your day with meditation and prayer. Ask for divine intervention in your choices throughout the day. When you are up against choices, i.e. what to eat or not to eat, getting your walking shoes on, or choosing water instead of another beverage to drink, tap into your spiritual resources.

G. **PASSION:** Enthusiasm, or passion, comes from the Greek word "pathos" meaning "in God," or in touch with the energy of the divine, so that you are filled with God's energy as it flows through your body. When you're in touch with that energy, you're alive. Today we use enthusiasm to describe fervent interest in things such as sporting events, and we've neglected the divine meaning of the word. However, as indicated in this chapter, this divine meaning is returning. Wouldn't it be nice to see the same passion for the National Day of Prayer in the spring as we have for the Super Bowl game?

H. GUARD THE TEMPLE: Your body is the temple of the Holy Spirit. (Corinthians 3:16-17) Your body was not designed to sit behind the computer hours on end, breathe polluted air, drink alcohol, eat "junk foods" with little nutritional value, pop pills to cure headaches caused by stress, use addictive substances, and stay awake long hours. When you take care of your body, you glorify your Maker!

WHAT IF TOMORROW NEVER COMES?

If I knew it would be the last time
I would be there to share your day,
well I'm sure you'll have so many more
so I can let just this one slip away.

For surely there's always tomorrow
to make up for an oversight,
and we always get a second chance
to make everything right..

There will always be another day
to say our, "I love you's"
and certainly there's another chance
to say our "Anything I can do's"

But just in case I might be wrong,
and today is all I get,
I'd like to say how much I love you
and I hope we never forget.

Tomorrow is not promised to anyone,
young or old alike,
and today may be the last chance
you get to hold your loved one tight.

So if you're waiting for tomorrow,
why not do it today?

— Author Unknown

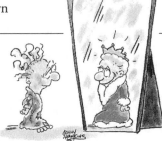

"Your life doesn't belong to you. Do what you can do today and don't wait for tomorrow, because tomorrow may never come."

— Enrique Perez, 107 years old

"Your body is the temple of the Holy Spirit."

— Corinthians 3:16-17

I once heard Zig Ziglar ask the audience if anyone owned a million dollar thoroughbred race horse. Of course no one did, but I could relate to what he was saying because we used to raise Morgan show horses and I knew the treatment we gave them. He asked,

> *If you had a valuable animal, would you leave it standing for days in the stall, feed it poor oats and spoiled hay, neglect the yearly shots and vet checks, neglect the regular 4-6 week hoof trimming and shoe replacement, fail to provide adequate water, and after a strenuous workout, put the horse away all sweated up?*

Obviously not. Everyone would do whatever had to be done to protect the health of a prize animal. Probably no one has that million dollar horse, but everyone has a million dollar body. Why then, does one do all the things to his/her body that he/she wouldn't do to a horse?

You have a responsibility to take care of your human temple. It is not the responsibility of your government, your physician, or anyone else. It is YOUR responsibility. By failing to treat your body with respect, you are dishonoring your Creator!

WHERE THE MIND GOES, THE BODY FOLLOWS

"The body is the temple of life. Energy is the force of life. If one of them goes off balance, all three are damaged. When the spirit takes command, the body naturally follows it. and this arrangement benefits all three treasures. When the body leads the way, the spirit goes along, and this harms all three treasures."

— Wen-Tzu, Ancient Chinese philosopher

WAYS TO GET SPIRITUAL

1. Healthy Lifestyle:

As we saw in Corinthians 3:16-17, your body is a temple. The connection goes like this: a healthy body creates a healthy mind; a healthy body and a healthy mind create a healthy spirit. Embrace wholeness. You are a physical, mental, and spiritual person. According to Larry Dossey, M.D., "You can't have a fit body if it's completely divorced from the mind and spirit." (Dossey)

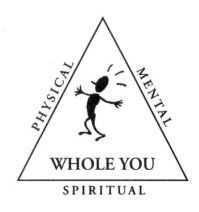

2. Awaken to Your Spiritual Needs:

Get passionate about your quest for God. An ancient Chinese proverb says, "When the student is ready, the teacher will appear." A Bible saying along the same lines is, "When you seek me, you will find me, when you search for me with all your heart." As your spiritual life grows, your passion for life will grow. Spiritual people filter their life events through their spiritual values. A passionate spiritual life can make all the difference in the world.

3. Go to the Book:

Find a book that complements your spiritual values. For many people, that will be the Bible. However, for others it might be the Koran or something similar. If it is an ancient book, try to find a newer version that is easier to read and understand.

4. Get Out in Nature:

Go for walks in the park, forest, by the lake or ocean. Get up early in the morning and watch the sunrise or watch the beauty of the sunset. Marvel at the birth of spring flowers or the wildlife that God has so abundantly provided. God's handprints are all over nature. "Be still and know that I am God." (Psalm 46:10)

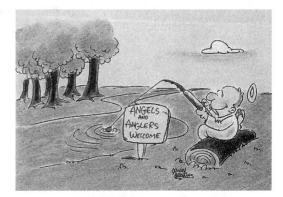

INDIAN SAYING

"Take time to see the sky,
Find shapes in the clouds,
Hear the murmur of the wind,
And touch the cool water,
Walk softly,
We are the intruders,
Tolerated briefly,
In our infinite Universe."

— Montezuma National Park, AZ

5. Prayer:

The word prayer comes from the Latin "precari," which means to entreat or ask earnestly, beseech, or implore. Prayer is a non-local event. It is not confined to a specific place in space or a specific moment in time. Prayer has many forms. It may be individual or communal, private or public. It may be offered in words, sighs, gestures, or silence. It may come from the conscious mind or from the depths of the unconscious.

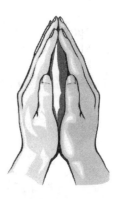

SAYING GRACE IN DIFFERENT RELIGIONS

"Let us give Thanks." "Bless us, O Lord, and these Thy gifts, which we are about to receive from Thy bounty. Through Christ our Lord. Amen" — **CATHOLIC.**

"O Christ our God, bless the food and drink of Thy servants. For Thou art Holy always, now and ever and unto ages of ages. Amen." — **ORTHODOX**

"Bless, O Lord, this food to our use, and us to Thy service, and make us ever mindful of the needs of others, in Jesus name. Amen." — **PROTESTANT**

"Lift up your hands toward the sanctuary and bless the Lord. Blessed are Thou, O Lord our God, King of the universe, who bringest forth bread from the earth. Amen." — **JEWISH**

"Everyone prays in their own language
and there is no language that God does not understand."

— Duke Ellington, famous musician

247

Studies show that prayer can have health benefits, regardless whether the praying person is in the presence of the person being prayed for or far away. Cardiologist Randolph Byrd conducted a study with patients who were prayed for in a coronary care unit at the San Francisco General Hospital. The study included 393 patients, 192 received prayer from a home prayer group, and 201 did not receive prayer. The study was a double-blind study, meaning that neither the patients, nurses, or doctors knew who was receiving prayer. The prayed-for-group had five times less need for antibiotics and were three times less likely to develop pulmonary edema. No one in the prayed-for-group needed an artificial airway, whereas 12 in the not-prayed-for group did. There were less deaths in the prayed-for-group. "If this technique had been a new drug or surgical procedure, it would have been considered a breakthrough in medicine." (Dossey 78)

Dr. Dale Matthews, a professor of medicine at Georgetown University, prays with patients who indicate a spirituality interest. However, he is still in the minority, as most physicians are reluctant to bring up the subject of religion with their patients. Dr. Matthews says, "It's almost never brought up in the doctors' office, even though it is very important to many people. Religion is the big elephant in the room that no one talks about."

Prior to writing his book, Healing Words, Dr. Larry Dossey was skeptical about the power of prayer. After his ten year study on prayer and spirituality, he has become a believer in praying for his patients. In his book, he reports the research and concludes saying, "Over time I decided that not to employ prayer with my patients was the equivalent of deliberately withholding a potent drug or surgical procedure. Never once did I pray for specific outcomes-for cancers to go away, for heart attacks to be healed, for diabetes to vanish. 'May the best possible outcome prevail' was the strategy I preferred, not specifying what 'best' meant." (Dossey xix)

Rainbows

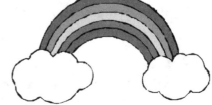

Rainbows appear after mighty storms,
When things look their very worst.
Just when skies are darkest gray,
Look for the rainbow first.

The rainbow is a sign of God's promise,
That He will guide us through all our trials.

No matter what their form,
When you feel battered by life's storms,
And you are filled with doubt and dismay,
Just remember God's rainbow will come,
For it's only a prayer away.

Does it matter HOW we pray? Some studies have shown that results occurred not only when people prayed for explicit outcomes, but also when they prayed for nothing specific. Some studies, in fact, showed a simple "Thy Will be Done," approach was more powerful than when specific results were held in the mind. I personally have found that "The Lord's Prayer" fits most occasions.

Does it matter WHEN we pray? For many, it means getting down on our knees, talking AND listening to God, i.e. saying grace before each meal, reciting verses during religious services, and saying prayers when tucking children into bed. For others, it is walking on the beach and noticing a beautiful sunset and saying simply, "Thank you Lord."

GET IN YOUR "PRAYER" CAR

For the following analogy of prayer, I'm indebted to Pastor Tamara Williams. Stevensville (MI) United Methodist Church

We use our car to get places, and in a similar way, we use prayer as a vehicle to get places.

- Prayers take us to God.

- Prayers take us places God wants us to go.

- Just like you have to put gas in your car, you have to put prayers in your body. Prayer is the fuel that gets us where we want to go. NOTE: The spiritual gas station is the church. Keep your tank filled.

- Prayers keep us fueled for the day. They give us help in getting to our places and through the day.

- We aren't the driver – God is the driver. Remember, "Thy will be done" not "my will be done." Prayer helps us to be aware of "Thy will." "Help me to fit in Your plan," not "You fit in my plan."

- Pray as often as you feel the need and wherever you feel the need, whether it's in the car, at work, while eating, or watching TV.

Get in your "prayer" car, so God can take you where He wants you to go. He has a great Master Plan for each of us.

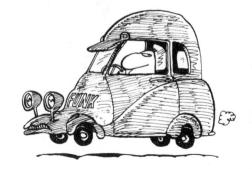

Americans are at a place in our culture where a lot of old boundaries are falling apart. The distinction between religious and secular is breaking down. Witness the changes in the workplace that have been discussed earlier. Never before have we had so many spiritual resources within easy reach. We are experiencing firsthand the values of meditation, massage, yoga, prayer, and many other forms of spiritual medicine.

"Spiritual involvement can get people in touch with an energy larger than themselves and that helps ease fear. For some, it might be attending a church service, for others taking a hike in the mountains or listening to beautiful music."
— Judith Orloff, author of Positive Energy

Spiritually, faith, prayer, religion - all mean different things to different people. No matter what the meaning, we are now beginning to uncover the healing potential of spirituality and the importance in connecting with a higher power.

There has always been a wellness hierarchy: the physical level, the emotional level, the intellectual level, and finally the spiritual level. For years we have been talking about the physical and emotional levels, and neglecting the spiritual level, but now we're starting to connect all the levels and, as we do, it can only improve the quality of life that we all so desperately seek.

BEST WISHES IN YOUR SPIRITUAL JOURNEY!

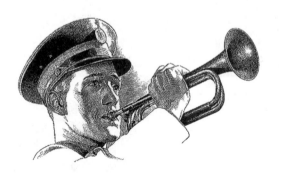

TAPS

Thanks and praise,
For our days,
'Neath the sun,
'Neath the stars,
'Neath the sky,
As we go,
This we know,
God is nigh.

(3rd verse of Taps)

CHAPTER THIRTEEN:
ENVIRONMENTAL

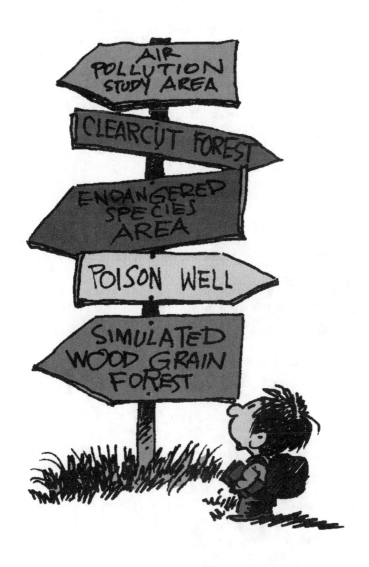

"Think Globally — Act Locally."

THE TOXIC ENVIRONMENT

It is no exaggeration to say that "Mother Earth" is in trouble. We have deforestation with the deliberate removal of trees, both in the tropics and our own country. Rain contains high concentrations of pollutants (acid rain). There is a debate whether global warming is fact or fiction. Air pollution is so bad that in some major cities, people are given ozone warnings to stay inside during certain periods of the day. We have ozone destruction which has resulted in greater exposure to ultraviolet rays, producing more cancers. Industrial chemicals are polluting the land, air, and water. Chemicals are in

> *We have a "throw-away" society! The average American generates 3.5 lbs of trash a day.*

our water supply. There are huge oil spills in our oceans. We are losing species of animals. We purchase vehicles that get 4-5 miles per gallon. Where I live on Lake Michigan, the water level has been down at least three feet for several years.

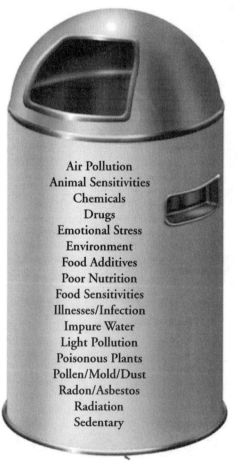

Air Pollution
Animal Sensitivities
Chemicals
Drugs
Emotional Stress
Environment
Food Additives
Poor Nutrition
Food Sensitivities
Illnesses/Infection
Impure Water
Light Pollution
Poisonous Plants
Pollen/Mold/Dust
Radon/Asbestos
Radiation
Sedentary

While industry contributes a major portion of pollutants to our land, air, and water, individual habits play a role as well. Our landfills overflow with packaging from our grocery and fast food purchases. We are accustomed to buying the latest model and discarding the old. We use vast quantities of plastic and paper products, disposable diapers, and Styrofoam.

Despite all these problems, and make no mistake they are serious problems, we fail to take responsibility for our actions. If you've been reading the previous chapters, you know that I'm a strong advocate of "individual" responsibility.

GARBAGE CAN OF ENVIRONMENTAL STRESSORS

Dr. Ruth Etzel, a leading pediatric environmental health expert, says, "We as Americans tend to take our environment for granted. Americans somehow have the notion that little decisions they make every day don't matter. Whether you choose to walk or drive your SUV to the grocery store four blocks away DOES matter. There's a saying that no snowflake in an avalanche ever feels responsible."

> *"The earth doesn't belong to us ... we belong to it."* — Chief Seattle

THINGS YOU CAN DO
TO HELP THE ENVIRONMENT

1. Don't run water unnecessarily.
2. Reduce waste.
3. Limit use of chemical pesticides.
4. Lower the thermostat.
5. Limit the use of air conditioners.
6. Install water saving devices.
7. Have an energy audit of your house.
8. Recycle.
9. Limit sprinkling/washing car.
10. Car pool to work.
11. Eat more fruits and vegetables and less meat.
12. Get involved.
13. Use public transportation.
14. Use fuel efficient cars.
15. Join an environmental action group.
16. Turn the lights off.
17. Visit and support our National Parks.
18. Buy wisely.
19. Keep tires inflated to improve gas mileage and extend tire life.
20. Organize a community group to clean beach, streets and highway.

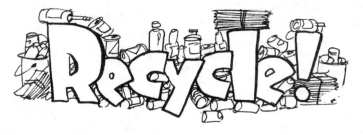

ALLERGIES

As a result of these environmental stressors, some people have immune systems that over-react and perceive what may be harmless to one individual as a threat to their body, producing an environmental illness commonly referred to as an allergy. The trigger, which is a protein to which the body reacts, is called an allergen. The allergens can be from foods, inhalants, chemicals, drugs, insects, or plants.

More than 60 million Americans suffer from allergenic conditions. Approximately 5,000 people die annually from asthma. Some 26 million cases of allergenic rhinitis (hay fever) is reported each year. Over 5 million U.S. school children are affected by asthma and about 15% of the population suffers from food allergies. More than 2 million are allergic to stinging insects.

The allergic person is often dramatically affected by minute quantities of a substance, whereas even large amounts of the same allergen cause no adverse reactions in non-allergic people. Penicillin is a good example. For most people, it heals by killing bacteria. However, a small group of people overreact to penicillin and this can be deadly.

About 16 million Americans have asthma. This translates to 7.5 percent of the American population. Between 1980 and 2002, the percentage has gone from three percent to 7.5 percent! While asthma has no known cause, some theories link it to diet and air pollution.

ALLERGENS

- **Foods** — peanuts, shell fish, spoiled fish (histamine), eggs, milk (lactose intolerance), wheat (gluten), corn, chocolate, beans, soy
- **Food additives** — acacia gum, benzoic acid, BHA, iron salts, MSG, propyl gallate, food coloring agents such as yellow dye no. 5, sulfites
- **Air Pollution**
- **Tissue Swelling** — hives

- **Contact Dermatitis** — poison ivy, poison oak, cosmetics, latex rubber
- **Insects** — bees, wasps, hornets, yellow jackets, fire ants
- **Drugs** — penicillin, sulfa, aspirin, ibuprofen
- **Chemicals** — those found in plastics and paints
- **Inhalants** — pollen from trees, weeds, grasses

The areas that we experience the most problems are the outside, the home, and workplace. The allergy picnic shown here has twenty potential allergens.

THE ALLERGY PICNIC

QUESTION: How many allergens can you identify? (Answers Below)

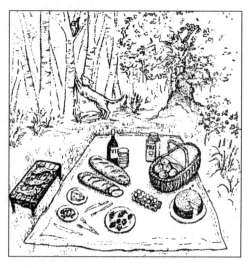

Cheese, milk, chocolate, eggs, tomatoes, bees, wine, wheat, peanut butter, fish, shrimp, dog/cat dander, oak/birch trees, timothy grass, plantain grass, bluegrass, poison oak/ivy.

THE TOXIC HOUSE

According to the Environmental Protection Agency (EPA), indoor air can be more polluted than the air on a busy street. In some areas, common household products, such as cleaners and cosmetics, are second only to the automobile as a source of air pollution. According to the EPA, "…we are actually poisoning ourselves in our homes and workplace everyday."

The Household Products Database, maintained by the National Library of Medicine, links more than 4,000 household products. Products range from air fresheners to weed killer. Sometimes answers can mean peace of mind and save a trip to the emergency room. Do a search for "Household Products Database."

QUESTION: How toxic is your house?

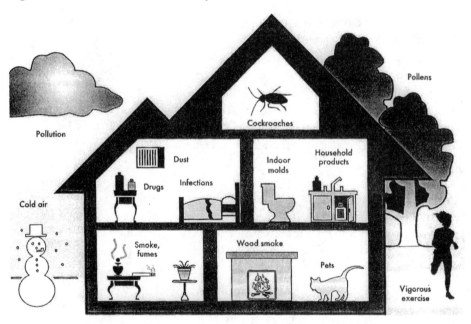

ENVIRONMENTAL TOXINS

Food Sensitivities	Air Pollution	Animal Sensitivities
Emotional Stresses	Lack of Exercise	Foods
Food Additives	Impure Water	Illnesses/Infection
Pollen/Mold/Dust	Chemicals	Radiation
Radon/Asbestos	Drugs	Plants
	Television/Computer Usage	

TREATMENT OF ENVIRONMENTAL TOXINS

Treatment involves the identification and blocking of these toxins before they produce severe reactions. While it is generally a slow and sometimes tedious process, there are many new medicines out there. In general, allergy treatment typically includes identification of the allergen (for avoidance), medications, and if necessary, allergy shots to diminish the frequency and intensity of future events.

You should see a doctor if you notice recurring symptoms or if you've had a severe reaction after exposure to an allergen. Even if you recover fully, future events could be catastrophic. Not only do you need regular medical follow-ups, but you also should always carry emergency medication and identification with you. This is extremely important.

I'll never forget the time I was teaching my college tennis class and one of my older students was stung by bees. The tennis courts were at a distance from the college, which was located several miles from the nearest medical facility and it was before the use of cell phones. She had perfume on (which she admitted later that was a no-no) which attracted the bees. Fortunately, she carried medicine with her which prevented a life threatening anaphylactic shock.

If your medical history suggests allergies, your doctor will likely recommend testing. The most common is skin testing which involves injecting tiny amounts of allergens under the skin and watching for an allergic response. Some doctors will instead use a blood test, called a RAST or radioallergosorbent test to evaluate the presence of antibodies associated with specific allergies.

SOURCES FOR ALLERGY HELP

- American Academy of Allergy and Immunology — 800-822-ASMA
- American Academy of Environmental Medicine — 316-684-5500
- American Environmental Health Foundation — 800-428-2343
- American College of Allergy, Asthma & Immunology — 847-427-1200
- National Asthma Education and Prevention Program (NIH) — www.nhlbi.nih.gov/about/naepp/index.htm
- The Food Allergy Network — 800-929-4040

CULTURAL FACTORS THAT CAN CAUSE THESE DISEASES

Physical Inactivity	Obesity	Television
Hypertension	Smoking	Cancer
Fast foods/Junk foods	Diabetes	Illegal Drugs
Osteoporosis	Excessive Alcohol	Arthritis

We fail to take responsibility for our actions. While we must "think globally" and be strong advocates of honoring "Mother Earth" by promoting approaches and attitudes that have long term solutions and not short term economic gains, we must "act locally." We can start with the little everyday decisions that we make as we go through our daily routines.

A few years ago, I went to a public hearing about whether a train carrying ore from a mine should be allowed to pass through an urban area twice a day, once to the mines and then back to the refinery. One mother with young children got up and spoke about how she didn't want her children exposed to the air pollution of the train passing her house. As she was leaving the meeting with her children, I observed her lighting up a cancer-ette. I asked her if she wasn't concerned about her kids inhaling the smoke. There was no answer.

Throughout the day and night, the average American is exposed to chemicals in his/her food, household cleaners, fumes of gasoline, pollutants in the air, and minute contaminants in the water. However, these risks pale in comparison to the risks one willingly assumes every day in using the automobile, smoking cancer-ettes , inappropriately using drugs and alcohol, failing to exercise and making inappropriate food choices.

Several studies have estimated that maybe as high as 32,000 Americans will die each year from environmental pollutants, food additives, industrial products, and occupational exposures. This pales to the 120,000 deaths from cancer-ette smoking, the 140,000 deaths associated with diet, and the 125,000 deaths from choosing to be sedentary. This is a total of almost 400,000 lifestyle deaths. These behaviors are all choices we have "chosen."

"Not to choose is to choose."

— Albert Camus, French philosopher

In the 1980's Kelly Brownell, a noted author and researcher on weight, came out with the conclusion that heredity was the controlling factor in weight control. This was based on a study of identical twins raised in different environments. However, in the early 1990's I attended a conference in Orlando, Florida, in which he had changed his viewpoint and now felt that while heredity was a factor, it was not the controlling factor. The dominant factor is the "toxic environment." He pointed out how our society is bombarded with ads on TV, billboards, and other media to enjoy the "good" life. He even predicted that in a few years we would see lawsuits against the fast food industry. At the time, I thought it would never happen. Unfortunately, this prediction has come true. We now have people refusing to put the blame where it belongs, on themselves, and trying to blame others for their poor choices.

The statistics are staggering. Over 60 percent of the population is overweight, only 20 percent of the population does the recommended physical activity of 30-60 minutes, six days a week, and over 50 percent of our meals are eaten away from our homes. We have become a "Super Sized" society. We have gallon jars of Miracle Whip, 50 oz. boxes of Frosted Flakes, 64 oz. "Double Gulps." Our cars are "Super Sized" as we've gone from the Explorer to the Expedition to the mammoth Excursion. Our adjectives of jumbo, mega, super, maxi, and extra value are commonplace.

As I've alluded to on many occasions in this book, we have taken movement out of our life! The body was designed by our Creator to MOVE, not sit on the sofa or in the computer for hours on end. The TV remote control has added 5 - 7 lbs per year to our body. The average person watches 4 hours a day of TV. During the course of a day, a person used to get up at least 15 times to change channels, raise/lower the volume, and turn it off and on, etc. Now a person turns on the TV, changes channels, answers the portable phone, mutes the TV, drinks a refreshment, etc. without leaving his/her overstuffed, self massaging, Lazy Boy chair. The same thing goes for the garage door opener, word processor, automatic transmission, riding lawn mower, leaf blower, snow blower, golf cart, cell phone and the list goes on.

WE TRULY HAVE A "TOXIC" ENVIRONMENT!

- WHAT CHANGES ARE YOU MAKING?
- YOUR CHOICES DO MAKE A DIFFERENCE!
- REMEMBER, IF IS TO BE, IT IS UP TO ME!

CHAPTER FOURTEEN:
COMPLEMENTARY AND ALTERNATIVE MEDICINE

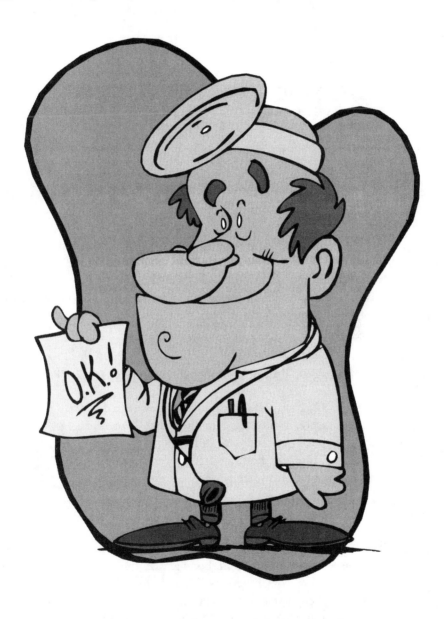

CLEAN BILL OF HEALTH

> *A significant amount of what we spend in health care is preventable. The public must play a part in making prudent decisions that will affect the quality of their lives and thereby decrease the cost. Examples would be ...obesity, diabetes, all of these are very much controllable if people make healthier decisions. I think everybody has to accept some responsibility to fix the system."*
>
> — Richard Carmona, 17th U.S. Surgeon General, 2003

COMPLEMENTARY AND ALTERNATIVE MEDICINE (CAM)

"Alternative," "natural," "holistic," "non-traditional," or "complementary" all refer to medicine that is thousands of years old. All are radically changing the American health care system.

No longer is the link of mind-body questioned. The traditional Western model of the body as a machine/robot has undergone a major overhaul. We have the proof of the effects of diet on cardiovascular health, the psychological boost we get from endorphins when we exercise, the stress-reduction that occurs in the presence of meditation, and the effects of healing with certain herbs, acupuncture and supplements.

DISEASE AS VIEWED BY CONVENTIONAL (WESTERN) AND COMPLEMENTARY (EASTERN) MEDICINE

WESTERN MEDICINE: Each part of the body is considered a distinct and separate entity, largely unconnected to the other. The heart, brain, and body are treated separately by different practitioners. I have experienced this problem first hand. There are certain conditions that I discuss with my family doctor, some with my orthopedic surgeon, others with my urologist, and still others with the cardiologist.

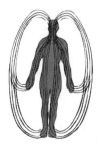

INTEGRATIVE MEDICINE: This concept views the body as a whole entity. Mind, body and spirit are all connected. The practitioner of Chinese medicine, the herbalist, the acupuncturist, or the chiropractor looks at the whole person from head to toe, physically and emotionally, when treating any condition.

COMPLEMENTARY MEDICINE + CONVENTIONAL = INTEGRATIVE MEDICINE

Ideally, Integrative Medicine employs the knowledge of modern science (i.e. Western medicine) without being constrained by it. As one proponent says, "If we do it correctly, we'll have one health system instead of two and healers of every stripe will work together."

In 1998, Congress established the National Center for Complementary and Alternative Medicine (NCCAM) at the National Institutes of Health (NIH). The primary mission of NCCAM is to provide the American public with reliable information about the safety and effectiveness of complementary and alternative medicine (CAM). Their budget quickly went from 2 million a year to over 100 million. They have many studies underway that will impact our health system.

COMPLEMENTARY AND ALTERNATIVE MEDICINE

ALTERNATIVE MEDICAL SYSTEMS
- Ayurvedic (Indian)
- Chiropractic
- Homeopathic
- Native American
- Naturopathic
- Traditional Chinese Medicine (acupuncture, Chinese herbal medicine)
- Environmental
- Osteopathic

MIND-BODY INTERVENTIONS
- Meditation
- Prayer and Mental Healing (visualization, imagery)
- Hypnosis
- Dance Therapy
- Art Therapy
- Music Therapy
- Humor

BIOLOGICAL BASED THERAPIES
- Special Diets (vegetarianism, macrobiotics, low carbohydrate)
- Aromatherapy
- Supplementation (vitamins, herbs)
- Biofeedback
- Exercise

MANIPULATIVE AND BODY BASED THERAPIES
- Massage (Swedish, sports, deep tissue, Shiatsu)
- Therapeutic Touch (body recall, touch for health, healing touch)
- Acupressure, Japanese Shiatsu (a variation of acupressure)
- Physical Therapy
- Reflexology
- Jin Shin Jyutsu (Japanese healing art)

ENERGY THERAPIES
- Tai Chi
- Yoga
- Pilates
- Magnets
- NIA (Neuromuscular Integrative Action)
- Qigong

This listing of CAM medicine is not a comprehensive list. A search of the field identified over 60 CAM systems that I haven't mentioned. For additional information contact the Office of Alternative Medicine (800-531-1794, 888-644-6226 or www.nccam.nih.gov.

CAM medicine is gaining more and more in acceptance. According to the National Institute of Health, over half of all Americans have used some kind of the above interventions, such as herbal remedies, massage, magnet therapy, acupuncture, and energy therapies. When you include vitamins, dietary interventions, and chiropractic treatment, the number of Americans using CAM approaches 100%. We make more visits to "non-conventional" healers (600 million a year) than we do to medical physicians. Total out of pocket spending on alternative medicine will top 50 billion dollars in 2001. This is more than will be spent on "traditional" hospital treatments.

One big problem is that the nation's insurers, including Medicare, are strongly biased against reimbursement of CAM therapies. All of the insurers fund bypass surgery at $50,000-$100,000 a surgery, but only a handful reimburse for Dr. Dean Ornish's lifestyle program which costs only $5,000 or even Dr. Hans Diehl's Coronary Health Improvement Program (CHIP) which is a bargain at less than $500.

As Dr. Andrew Wiel, MD, one of the leading proponents of CAM, says, "If I have alarming symptoms that indicate disease in a vital organ, symptoms stronger than I've had before, or symptoms that last for a longer time, I will seek a standard medical evaluation. For other conditions, I want to see if lifestyle changes, such as dietary, herbal, or relaxation will work. In other words, I want to let the body have a chance to heal itself."

"Even in China, no one says, 'Get me to an herbalist' after a car crash," says Dr. David Eisenberg, director of Harvard's Medical School for CAM. Thus, I would like to advance what is viewed by many as the ideal medical system, i.e. an integration of complementary and conventional medicine into integrative medicine.

Unfortunately, we have been conditioned to depend on drugs and medical procedures to fix symptoms without any thought to the personal power we possess to create and maintain our own health. Remember, "If it is to be, it is up to ME!"

Richard Samat, MD says, "Always start with the least morbid, least invasive treatment with the fewest side effects. This may mean trying non-traditional, non-pharmaceutical therapies like massage, spinal manipulation, acupuncture, and herbal first, instead of the other way around."

The accepted definition of CAM is any therapy that is not accepted by the dominant medical establishment in a given culture. Therefore, in China many medical procedures that we view as mainstream, such as the use of medication to control arthritis, cancer, and heart disease would be viewed as alternative.

In the Western hemisphere, the advocates of alternative and traditional medicine have often been at loggerheads. Alternative medicine advocates view conventional doctors as so focused on disease or body parts that they have no compassion for the whole person. They are viewed as money-loving individuals, in partnership with the drug companies, and out to take the patient's life savings. The medical advocates view alternative medicine as unproven, worthless, dangerous, and steeped in anecdotal (non scientific) case histories.

Obviously, the truth is somewhere in the middle. While it is true that there is a scarcity of scientific evidence to support the claims to healing made by proponents of alternative medicine, that is due more to how research is funded than to the merits of each approach. Drugs are not developed simply to ease pain and suffering. The issue of money (profits) is always involved. Pharmaceutical companies spend millions of dollars on research so they can have a patent worth billions. Why would they want to spend millions on the effectiveness of St John's Wort when they can't patent an already discovered drug and make a profit from it? Aspirin is a classic example. If aspirin were discovered today, it would cost mega bucks for a jar of 50 capsules, instead of $3.95.

A COMPARISON OF CAM
AND WESTERN MEDICINE

CAM is strongest in areas where Western medicine is weakest, namely chronic illnesses such as arthritis, sleep problems, back pain, and heart disease. These areas are the strengths of the Traditional Chinese Medical System. At the risk of oversimplification, the following illustration shows the differences on how the Western trained physician and the Chinese doctor will treat the patient who has sleep problems.

CHINESE MEDICINE: The patient will be prescribed acupuncture, Qigong (Chinese yoga), meditation, dietary modifications, herbal remedies, and possibly feng shui (pronounced fung schway) which is the room arrangement to maximize the flow of Qi or life energy that is always present. In other words, the patient will be given a major lifestyle change.

WESTERN MEDICINE: The scientific approach will include prescription drugs, if necessary a night in the sleep lab analyzing the sleep pattern, possibly a class in stress reduction, and dietary modifications.

The same analogy could be made for low back pain, arthritis, and many more chronic diseases. Wouldn't it be better to combine the two systems and get a synergistic effect, instead of the either or approach?

What draws many people to CAM is a desire to be cared for. People like to be talked to and touched. Tieraona Low Dog, MD says, "We need a health system that can do more than count." Though more medical schools offer courses in CAM, few of today's doctors have learned to go beyond the lab tests to see how the patient really feels.

The above is not intended to discredit traditional medical and pharmaceutical procedures. Personally, I have recently experienced some serious health problems (heart), and I'm truly thankful for the medical technology that has developed the pacemaker, the refinement of bypass surgery, and the development of the statin drugs to lower cholesterol. I'm also thankful for the simple aspirin, folate, and B complex vitamins that allow me to control the CRP and homocysteine factors that I've inherited. This is what I mean by integrative medicine.

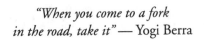

"When you come to a fork in the road, take it" — Yogi Berra

BE A RESPANT

As I outlined in Chapter 10, be a RESPANT — responsible participant. Don't continue to merely ask the practitioners of conventional and alternative medicine, "What do you recommend?" or "What do you think is best?" Instead ask, "What is the evidence that supports what you recommend?" We should investigate the pros and cons BEFORE putting the remedy in our body.

1. **CONSIDER THE RISKS.** Just because it's "natural" doesn't mean that it's harmless! An example is St. John's Wort, a "natural" herb that can interact badly with blood thinning drugs, such as aspirin and Coumadin.

2. **DON'T UNDERESTIMATE YOUR PROBLEM.** A back pain could be more than a pulled muscle.

3. **TALK OPENLY WITH YOUR DOCTOR.** Inform your doctor about ALL remedies you use. If your physician doesn't appear knowledgeable and open minded about CAM, maybe it's time to find another medical provider. I have a philosophy, "You can't be down on something, you're not up on." I would like my physician to be open minded.

PATIENTS NOT GETTING ENOUGH FITNESS/WEIGHT ADVICE
Primary-care physicians aren't addressing their patients' fitness and weight levels when they come in for check-ups. By adding three extra minutes on the patients' office visit, physicians could use their unique ability to discuss body mass index, counsel them on food intake, exercise and strength training. These three minutes could go a long way in reducing the 300,000 premature deaths and 90 billion dollars in health care costs attributed to lifestyle per year.

---

4. **DO YOUR HOMEWORK.** Check the authenticity of your sources. Be careful about information you find on the Web as there is a lot of erroneous information on it. For starting out, a good source is the National Center for Complementary and Alternative Medicine (www.nccam.nih.gov). Another source is The Alternative Medicine Association at 415-435-1779 or e-mail: editor@alternativemedicine.com.

PILATES, QIGONG, TAI CHI AND YOGA
JOIN WESTERN WELLNESS

Twenty years ago Pilates, Qigong, Tai Chi and Yoga were considered to be on the fringe of mainstream wellness. Those who practiced these ancient Chinese (Tai Chi and Qigong), Indian (Yoga), and American (Pilates) disciplines were viewed as "different." However, today these are the fastest growing classes in the health and fitness clubs. Advocates of Tai Chi, Yoga, and Qigong emphasize that they are NOT a religion, but a spiritual discipline that can coexist and reinforce any religion. This is a subtle, but important difference.

The theme throughout this book has been that mind, body, and spirit are interconnected. Wellness techniques that promote a deeper mind/body awareness have been practiced by Eastern cultures for thousands of years. It's only in the past few years that these programs have been accepted into Western medicine. Used as a form of fitness and health promotion these gently moving arts incorporate breathing exercises and deep relaxation with gentle movements.

QIGONG

Qigong (pronounced chi-gong) is a slow motion exercise that is older than Tai Chi. Qi means "life force or breath energy" and gong means "practice or skills." Qi is an intrinsic energy in the body that travels along pathways in the body called meridians. These are the same pathways where acupuncturists place needles to cure or alleviate a patient's conditions. The purpose is to restore the flow of qi to a natural, healthy balance. Today, Qigong is widely used in Chinese hospitals to speed the recovery of convalescent patients by opening up blocked energy pathways. For additional information on Qigong contact the YMAA Publishing Center, 4354 Washington St., Boston, Massachusetts 02131 (800-669-8892) www.ymaa.com@aol.com.

TAI CHI AND QIGONG IN THE 18 STYLE

There are literally thousands of forms of Qigong. I recently took a class which incorporated Tai Chi and Qigong into a program called "Tai Chi, Qigong in the 18 Style." I found this class very invigorating. It incorporates movements such as "Caressing a fountain," "Gazing from a mountaintop," "Wave hands like clouds," "Dancing with a rainbow," "Children bouncing a ball," "Waves in the ocean" and "Watching the train go by." The complete program of 18 gentle flowing movements takes about 3 minutes. I have put together a video tape in which the instructor Andy Green does each movement six times. The entire routine is 20 minutes, and serves as a great way to warm up before beginning the day.

If you desire additional information on "Tai Chi, Qigong in the 18 Style," contact Dahlis Roy at 269-556-1955 or e-mail: dahlis.roy@gte.net. For an instructor page go to www.sidekickstaekwondo.com.

TAI CHI

Tai Chi has been called "yoga in motion" or "moving meditation." Like all the other Eastern disciplines, Tai Chi assists in the strength building of core muscles, builds better balance, improves concentration and increases flexibility.

Tai Chi incorporates slow, flowing, continuous movements performed in circular motions, and focuses on breathing and balance. It does not involve high-impact movements like running or jumping. It is used to encourage relaxation, reduce stress, and promote the circulation of "chi" or life energy within the body.

For additional information on Tai Chi contact, Dr. Paul Lam, MD at www.taichiproductions. com. Dr. Lam is a gold medallist in Tai Chi competition and a world authority in Tai Chi and Qigong. He has many videos and books, one of these being a video and book on "Tai Chi for Arthritis."

YOGA

Yoga is a form of exercise, and a method of attaining a higher state of consciousness through proper breathing and meditation. The exercise is performed through quiet, powerful stretching. The higher state of consciousness is accomplished through focused breathing and creative visualization. Yoga means to harmonize or unite the body, mind, and spirit so they work together.

> *"As long as there is breath in the body, there is life. When breath departs, so too does life. Therefore, regulate the breath."*
>
> — *Hatha Yoga Pradipika*

HATHA YOGA

Again, as with the other disciplines, there are many forms of physical yoga. Most of the yoga practiced by over 20 million Americans is a form known as Hatha or Western Yoga. "Ha" means sun and "tha" means moon. Hatha Yoga is known as the "yoga of force" which emphasizes strengthening and purifying the body. Hatha is actually an umbrella term that encompasses many varieties. Some of them are Ashtanga (power yoga), Bikram (hot yoga), Kupalu, Iyengar, and Viniyoga yogas. (body alignment through poses).

For yoga information: Yoga Intel. (800-253-6243), Yoga Journal (800-436-9642).

PILATES

Pilates (pronounced "pea-lot-eez) is a newcomer to the fitness field but it has become one of the fastest growing fitness activities in the country. In 1997, only 10% of the fitness clubs were offering Pilates but this quickly rose to 47% in 2001.

For information on Pilates contact the Institute for the Pilates Method at 800-505-1990. Another source is The Pilates Body, by Brook Siler.

ALTERNATIVE MEDICINE: NEVER BE DOWN ON SOMETHING YOU'RE NOT UP ON

I recently attended a health conference where the speaker said that she had a rule to "never be down on something you're not up on." Even the American Medical Association is willing to give the benefit of the doubt. Many alternative therapies that are now considered mainstream were rejected just a few years ago.

In order to be up on alternative medicine, you could read The Guide To Holistic Health, edited by Larry Trivieri. This book is a comprehensive overview of 20 major disciplines of holistic medicine, including acupuncture, ayurvedic medicine, bodywork, chiropractic, environmental medicine, naturopathy, osteopathy, traditional Chinese medicine, and yoga. Most importantly, this is the first book endorsed by the American Holistic Medical Association.

POGO says, "We have met the enemy — he is us"

ALTERNATIVE MEDICINE GOES "MAINSTREAM"

According to a nationwide survey, 36 percent of adults use some form of complementary and alternative medicine, or CAM. The 10 most commonly used therapies and the approximate percentage of U.S. adults using each therapy were:

Prayer for own health	43%
Prayer by others	24%
Natural products	13%
Deep breathing exercises	12%
Group prayer	10%
Meditation	8%
Chiropractic care	8%
Yoga	5%
Massage	5%
Diet-based therapies (Atkins, Pritikin, Ornish)	4%

SOURCE: Centers for Disease Control and Prevention

CHAPTER FIFTEEN:
INTEGRATIVE MEDICINE: BRINGING IT TOGETHER

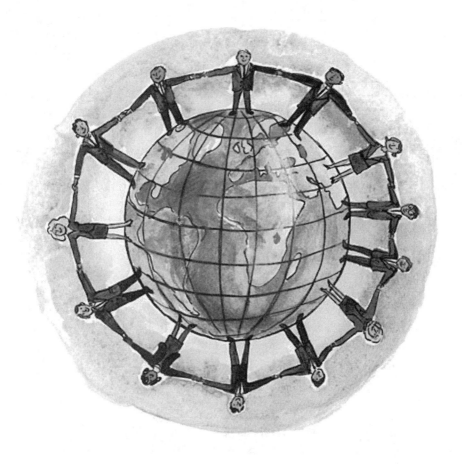

*"It's easier to maintain your health
than it is to regain it once you've lost it."*

— Kenneth Cooper, MD

EASTERN AND WESTERN MEDICINE MEET

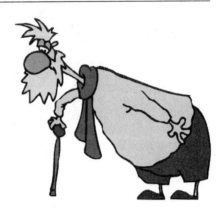

"If I had known I was going to live this long, I'd have taken better care of myself."

— Eubie Blake
(Feb. 7, 1883-Feb. 12, 1983)

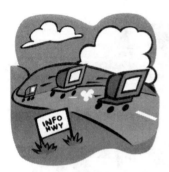

At the beginning of the book, I asked you to come with me down the wellness path. Now, you've traveled with me through these 250 plus pages, I hope that you've learned more about wellness than you knew when you started. I know that I have. Initially, when I started this project of revising the book I'd written several years ago, I thought that it would be a quick and easy task. How wrong I was! Of course, having the heart attack and related problems during this span didn't help things, but that aside, I was amazed at how much about wellness had changed in just two years. Every day there is new information about nutrition, supplementation, fitness, etc., but there is one thing that has not changed and NEVER will. That is, if you want to enjoy good health, it's up to you! No one can do it for you! I struggle with that at times, and when I falter, I know that I'm to blame, not the environment or my genes. The sad part is that we now have more knowledge about our bodies than at any time in our history, but we still continue to abuse them. We know what we should do, BUT we don't do it.

The theme of this book has been the integration of conventional (Western) medicine with complementary (integrative) medicine. I've tried to highlight the best of both worlds so that as Dr. Hans Diehl says, "You can truly live the 'good' life. The one that our creator has intended for all of us."

HOW LONG MIGHT YOU LIVE?

It's never too late to change bad habits that could shave years off your life. If you would like to live to be 100, take the online quiz developed by the Alliance for Aging Research, based on the New England Centenarian Study. (www.beeson.org)

WELLNESS TERMINOLOGY

Many times we use the words complementary, integrative, and alternative interchangeably. However, there are subtle distinctions among the three terms.

COMPLEMENTARY: *means that the treatment is intended to be used in addition to the standard proven treatment option, i.e. to complement what we already know works.*

INTEGRATIVE: *means that the treatment is designed to work together, i.e. a blending of traditional and non-traditional treatment.*

ALTERNATIVE: *means that the treatment is to be used instead of known and accepted treatments.*

The term "alternative" should raise a red flag. Often, it is unproven treatment. By using this, you face two serious problems: first, the treatment may not work and the disease will continue, thus you've lost valuable time, and secondly, the treatment may actually be dangerous and cause you harm.

In my opinion, the key is to integrate and/or complement the treatment options. This gives you the maximum chance for optimum health.

HOLISTIC MEDICAL MODEL

To summarize everything you've read, I'm going to rely on my friend and respected internist, Roger L. Greenlaw, MD of Rockford, Illinois, to put everything in perspective. On a recent cruise, Roger and his wife Carolyn presented very interesting sessions on how you can combine the holistic or complementary field with the conventional field in aging gracefully. I've heard many speakers talk about this concept, but no one brought things into perspective as clearly as they did. What makes it all the more meaningful is that it's obvious that they "walk their talk." Both of them, while being in their late 50's, (I'm just guessing, but Roger has been a medical doctor for almost 30 years), lead a very active lifestyle and appear to be in excellent health.

Roger has become very active in the American Holistic Medical Association and has been successful in combining the best of the complementary and conventional. He is an officer in the Holistic Medical Association and also the medical advisor of the Coronary Health Improvement Program (CHIP), in addition to being head of the Internal Medicine Dept. at Swedish Covenant Hospital in Rockford.

In his workshop, Roger presented a Holistic Model for the Integration of the differing medical systems. If we could get our medical system on board, we could truly have one system, instead of two. Roger gives the credit for this concept to Elliott Dacher, MD who has authored a best seller on holistic medicine, <u>Whole Healing</u>.

In this book, Dr. Dacher, a Harvard trained physician, advocates an unconventional approach to healing. His "Whole Healing System" rests on four healing systems: homeostasis (an automatic, internal balancing system within our bodies), treatment (drugs, surgery, or alternative therapies), mind/body healing (growing from increased awareness), and spiritual healing (based on expansion of the consciousness). He shows how these four systems together have a remarkable power to keep us well. Through the use of "inner journeys," he shows how we can access these four systems simultaneously for renewed health. These "journeys" are based on more than twenty years of treating thousands of patients.

A HOLISTIC MEDICAL MODEL FOR CHRONIC DISEASE PREVENTION, ARREST AND REVERSAL

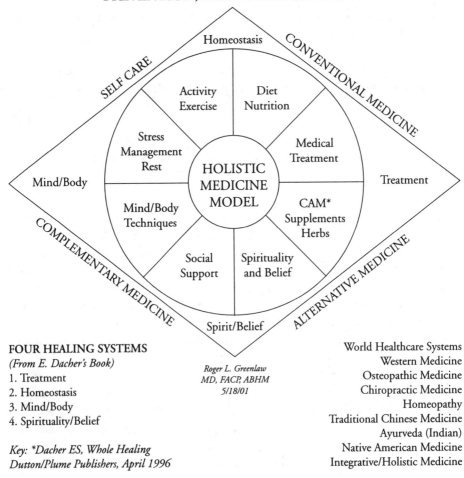

FOUR HEALING SYSTEMS
(From E. Dacher's Book)
1. Treatment
2. Homeostasis
3. Mind/Body
4. Spirituality/Belief

Roger L. Greenlaw
MD, FACP, ABHM
5/18/01

World Healthcare Systems
Western Medicine
Osteopathic Medicine
Chiropractic Medicine
Homeopathy
Traditional Chinese Medicine
Ayurveda (Indian)
Native American Medicine
Integrative/Holistic Medicine

*Key: *Dacher ES, Whole Healing*
Dutton/Plume Publishers, April 1996

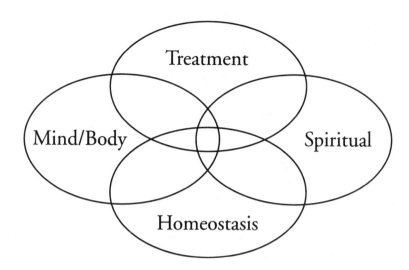

In this model, patients are encouraged to evaluate treatment of any medical or health issue by developing an approach to treatment that includes each area on the circle, i.e. medical treatment, diet/nutrition, activity/exercise, stress management skills/adequate rest, mind body techniques, social support, spirituality/belief, and complementary and alternative medicine supplements (herbal therapy, etc.). This approach will activate the four healing systems.

Using the Holistic Medical Model as a guide to treatment planning assures the greatest opportunity for healing that involves state of the art medical care (Eastern and conventional) and maximum empowerment of the patient in the area of self care.

IN OTHER WORDS, IT IS THE BEST OF BOTH WORLDS!

NOTE: View the Holistic Medicine Model for physicians at www.wholehealing.org.

KEEP YOUR PERSONAL HEALTH JOURNAL

We keep complete maintenance records for our cars with dates and details of each servicing. Do our bodies deserve anything less? I was just reading a wellness article in which the writer says, "I took better care of my dogs and car than myself." Sadly, that's not uncommon.

In the past, people often stayed with the same doctor for life and most medical records were in one place. Today, as I covered in previous chapters, we see many different doctors, each treating a different malady and we are a much more mobile society now. In addition, our health insurance often dictates that we change providers.

It is up to us as "respants" (responsible participants) to help coordinate our care. It is impossible for your doctor to know what other doctors have prescribed without you furnishing a complete list of prescribed medications, over the counter medicines, and vitamin and herbal supplements. Many doctors have several thousand patients. Most doctors request that you bring your medications with you at each visit. Lab test results and other data in a personal health journal may help your doctor to identify trends without having to duplicate tests. Having a health journal may save you money, frustration, and time by helping you track reimbursements and appeal denials by your insurance company. Enough reasons?

> **BE A RESPANT:** *There are 126 schools in the country that teach you how to be a physician, but not one for how to be a patient. Take charge of your care! (United Health Foundation — uhftips.org)*

My wife and I have compiled a list of all medications and surgeries on a computer. We keep a copy in our cars and with our medications. That way if we make an emergency trip to the hospital, we've got the information handy. I recently read about a person who was taken to the hospital by ambulance, and because his prescription listing wasn't handy, he was administered medication that conflicted with what he was taking.

Okay, how can you start a personal medical diary? Obviously, you can take a notebook and after each visit write down date, symptoms and diagnosis. However, printed medical diaries are available in bookstores or online. They simplify the whole process with separate sections for tracking medical visits, prescription drugs, blood pressure, cholesterol, and other important information.

Two choices are: The Lifetime Health Journal by Karolina Kawiaka, and Memory Minder: Personal Health Journal, by Frances Wilkins. Medical diaries are also available online without charge. One is the Personal Health Care Journal at www.aoa.gov@smp/journal.pdf.

GIFT SUGGESTION:

A journal can make a wonderful baby shower gift for expectant parents.
Parents can track the child's health and use the book to record significant events in the child's life. This could be the start of a life-long journal.

ASSEMBLE YOUR
PERSONAL WELLNESS TEAM

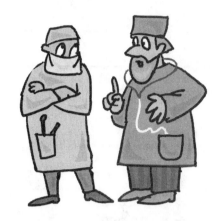

It is said that the amount of information at our disposal doubles every five years. With the Internet, it probably is less time than that. Therefore, I would suggest everyone consider assembling their personal wellness team. This team should be composed of traditional and non traditional specialists. Don't wait until you have a medical crisis to put this team together. Do it when you're healthy!

The composition of the team will vary, depending on your personal preferences and ideas about wellness. My wellness team will be different than yours and will continually change. It is important to have confidence in your wellness team. I have changed doctors because I didn't think my doctor was "walking the talk" when it came to lifestyle choices or keeping current with medical advances.

YOUR COMPREHENSIVE WELLNESS TEAM

PRIMARY DOCTORS (ESSENTIAL)

Medical Doctor: _____

Spiritual Doctor: _____

Nutritional Doctor (RD, ND): _____

Physical Fitness Doctor: _____

Pharmacist: _____

Hospital(s): _____

_____

Specialists (Orthopedics, Internists, Cardiologists, Podiatrists, etc)

_____

_____

_____

_____

ADDITIONAL "DOCTORS" THAT ARE NICE TO KNOW

Audiologist: _____

Acupuncturist:_____

Chiropractic/Osteopathic Doctor: _____

Herbalist: _____

Massage Therapist: _____

Naturopathic Doctor: _____

Personal Trainer: _____

Physical Therapist: _____

Stress Doctor: _____

Supplement Doctor: _____

Tai Chi, Yoga, Qigong, etc: _____

Veterinarian: _____

Other:_____

_____

_____

NOTE: Some of these people could fill two or three positions on your team. For example, an osteopathic doctor can do chiropractic manipulations. Many nutritionists also have expertise in physical fitness, supplements and herbs.

FOR A NATUROPATHIC PHYSICIAN (nutrition and supplementation), I would contact the American Association of Naturopathic Physicians at www.naturopathic. org, or 703-610-9037.

FOR A MASSAGE THERAPIST, obtain word-of-mouth recommendations from friends and then give them a personal trial. My personal rule is that if I can't see any improvement within 4-5 visits, it's usually time to look elsewhere for assistance.

FOR AN HERBALIST, you can contact the American Herbalistic Guild at www.healthy.net/herbalists. Many dietitians have experience with supplements, including herbs.

TO FIND A REGISTERED DIETITIAN (RD), you can contact the American Dietetic Association at www.eatright.org.

FOR A CHIROPRACTOR, you can contact the Chiropractic Licensing Board at www.fclb.org or get a referral from a friend.

TO LEARN MORE ABOUT THE EASTERN MODALITIES, SUCH AS ACUPUNCTURE, I would suggest the American Association of Acupuncture and Oriental Medicine at 202-265-2287.

FOR TAI CHI, YOGA, QIGONG, AND PILATES, I would contact your local fitness club, college, or wellness center. Most communities have at least one wellness center, and they are a great source for leading edge information.

NATIONAL WELLNESS INSTITUTE CONFERENCE

If you are seeking additional information about wellness, I would recommend attending the annual National Wellness Institute Conference in July at Stevens Point, WI. This is a 5-day gathering of 1,200-2,000 people interested in learning more about personal and work-site wellness. Contact the National Wellness Institute at 800-244-8922 or e-mail NWI@nationalwellness.org.

LATE BREAKING NEWS

Note: As this book was being prepared for publication, the American Academy of Family Physicians released a study on the future of American medicine. The possibilities that this model offers for medical treatment are mind boggling.

The lead researcher, Dr. James Martin, a family doctor and head of the American Academy of Family Physicians, says, "This is where the U.S. health care system needs to go." Dr. John Bucholtz, co-author of the study, hopes that the study will lead to a new system of care that benefits doctors and patients. "Otherwise, it's just a bunch of Band-Aids on a broke system."

The model has been endorsed by many groups, including the American Medical Association (AMA), American Academy of Pediatrics (AAP), American Association of Retired Personnel (AARP), Medicare, Blue Cross Blue Shield Association, and a trade group, the America's Health Insurance Plans.

Until it becomes operational, you should continue assembling your personal wellness team. When this plan becomes operational you will be ahead of the game.

CURRENT HEALTH CARE MODEL:

Treatment is centered around a visit to a primary care doctor who acts as a "gatekeeper" to health services.

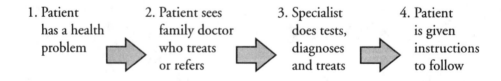

1. Patient has a health problem

2. Patient sees family doctor who treats or refers

3. Specialist does tests, diagnoses and treats

4. Patient is given instructions to follow

PROPOSED HEALTH CARE MODEL:

The patient and family doctor work together to make informed decisions. They are supported by many services and health professionals.

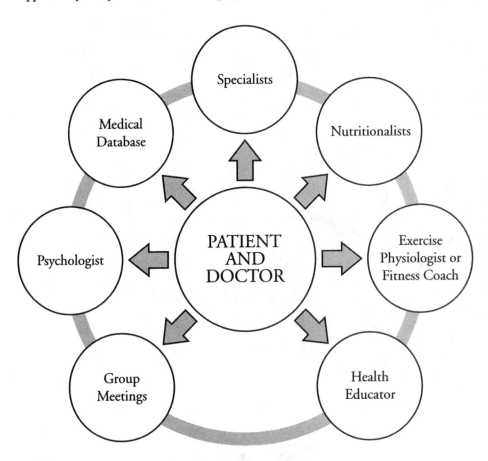

FEATURES OF THE "NEW" MEDICAL SYSTEM:

- Patients will schedule appointments online
- Patients will have online access to nurse educators and other medical specialists
- Patients will meet with nutritionists, psychologists and health coaches
- Patients can e-mail questions to their doctor or nurse
- Doctors will have access to national database of updated medical guidelines
- Doctors can share test results, X ray, and medications with specialists, pharmacists and hospitals

Source: The American Academy of Family Physicians. Released 03/30/04, San Antonio, TX

I'D RATHER SEE A SERMON
— Edgar A. Guest

I'd rather see a sermon

than hear one any day;

I'd rather one should walk with me

than merely show the way,

The eye's a better pupil,

And more willing than the ear;

Fine counsel is confusing,

But example's always clear.

I soon can learn to do it,

If you'll let me see it done;

I can see your hands in action,

But your tongue too fast may run;

And the lectures you deliver,

May be very fine and true;

But I'd rather get my lesson,

By observing what you do.

For I may misunderstand you,

And the high advice you give,

But there's no misunderstanding

how you act and how you live.

SUMMING IT UP:
WELLNESS IS A
LIFETIME COMMITMENT

COMPENSATION

I'd like to think when life is done
That I had filled a needed post,
That here and there I'd paid my fare
With more than idle talk and boast;
That I had taken gifts divine,
The breath of life and manhood fine
And tried to use them now and then
In service for my fellow men.

I'd hate to think when life is through
That I had lived my round of years
A useless kind that leaves behind
No record in this vale of tears;
That I had wasted all my days
By treading only selfish ways,
And that this world would be the same
If it had never known my name.

I'd like to think that here and there,
When I am gone, there shall remain
A happier spot that might have not
Existed had I toiled for gain;
That some one's cheery voice and smile
Shall prove that I had been worth while;
That I had paid with something fine
My debt to God for life divine.

— Edgar A. Guest

"You have the power to maintain your own health. It's up to you to take that responsibility. The choices you make and your habits are much more powerful than anything we in medicine can provide." — James Rippe, MD

It is my sincere desire that you have enjoyed this book and will pass it on to family and friends. Remember, wellness is a journey, not a destination. Heed the advice of Winston Churchill, "NEVER, NEVER, NEVER GIVE UP!"

When I was a youngster, I remember hearing someone say that your life has been a success if you can say that you left the earth in better shape than when you arrived. They went on to say that when you get to heaven they'll ask you whose life you made better by knowing you. So please do me a favor. After you've read this book, send me your success story so that when I get to the gates of heaven and I'm asked whose life I touched, I'll be able to give them your name.

Best wishes on your wellness journey,
— Don

The Old Irish Blessing

May the road rise to meet you;
May the wind be always at your back;
The sun shine warm upon your face,
The rains fall soft upon your fields,
And until we meet again,
May God hold you in the palm of his hands.

THE DASH

I read of a man who stood to speak
at the funeral of a friend.
He referred to the dates on her tombstone
from the beginning... to the end.
He noted that first came her date of birth
and spoke the following date with tears:
But he said what mattered most of all
was the dash between those years (1934-1998).
For that dash represents all the time
that she spent alive on earth...
And now only those who loved her know
what that little line is worth.
For it matters not, how much we own;
the cars... the house... the cash...
What matters is how we live and love
and how we spend our dash.
So think about this long and hard...
are there things you'd like to change?
For you never know how much time is left,
that can still be rearranged.
If we could just slow down enough
to consider what's true and real,
And always try to understand
the way other people feel
And be less quick to anger,
and show appreciation more
And love the people in our lives
like we've never loved before.
If we treat each other with respect,
and more often wear a smile....
Remembering that this special dash
might only last a little while.
So, when your eulogy's being read
with your life's actions to rehash...
Would you be proud of the things they say
about how you spent your dash?

— Anonymous

AARP Bulletin, Feb, 2004.

Alsbro, Donald, Ed.D.. The Best Little Book of Wellness, Benton Harbor, MI: Rainbow Wellness, 2000. 269-925-3524.

Annals of Pharmacotherapy, 2002, vol. 36, no. 12.

Archives of Internal Medicine, 9 July 2000.

Balch, James, M.D., Prescription for Nutritional Healing, 7th Edition, New York: Penquin Putnum, 2000.

Benson, Herbert, M.D., Timeless Healing, the Biology of Belief, New York: Dane Publishing, 1996.

Benson, Herbert, M.D., The Wellness Book, New York: Birch Lane Press, 1992.

Borysenko, Joan, Minding the Body, Mending the Mind, New York: Bantam, 1988.

Complete Book of Natural and Medicinal Cures, New York: Rodale Press, 1994.

Covey, Steven, Seven Habits of Highly Effective People, New York: Simon & Schuster, 1984.

Cousins, Norman, Anatomy of an Illness as Perceived by the Patient, New York: Bantom, 1979.

Dacher, Elliott, M.D., Whole Healing, New York: Dutton/Plume, 1996.

Diehl, Hans, Ph.D., Health Power: Health by Choice Not Chance, California: Review and Herald Publishing Association, 2000.

Dossey, Larry, M.D., Healing Words, New York: Harper, 1993.

Dossey, Larry, M.D., Reinventing Medicine, New York: Harper Collins, 1999.

Evans, William, Ph.D., Biomarkers, New York: Simon and Schuster, 1992.

Frankl, Victor, Man's Search for Meaning, Boston: Beacon Print, 2000.

Haebig, Jeff, Ph.D., Wellness Quest (series of books), Rochester, Minnesota: Wellness Quest, 1995.

Hendersen, Joe, editor, "Remembering George," Runner's World, Dec. 2003: 61.

Jacobson, Michael, Ph.D., and Jane Hurley, R.D., Restaurant Confidential, New York: Workman Publishing, 2000.

Jeffers, Susan, Feel the Fear and Do It anyway, New York: Random House, 1996.

Ludington, Aileen, M.D. and Hans Diehl, Ph.D., Dynamic Living, California: Review Herald Publishing Association, 2000.

Matthews, Dale, M.D., The Faith Factor: Proof of the Healing Power of Prayer, New York: Penquin Putnam, 1999.

Moses, Jeffrey, Oneness: Great Principles Shared by All Religions, New York: Fawcett Columbine, 1989.

New England Journal of Medicine, 2003, vol. 348, no. 26.

Prochaska, James O., Changing for Good, New York: Avon, 1994.

Rippe, James, M.D., New England Journal of Medicine, Boston:

Robertson, Robin, Vegan Planet, Boston: Harvard Common Press, 2003.

Roizen, Michael F., M.D., Real Age, New York: Cliff Street Books, 1999.

Roizen, Michael F., M.D., Real Age Makeover, New York: Harper, 2004.

Trivieri, Larry, editor, The Guide to Holistic Health, New York: John Wiley and Sons, 2001.

USA Today, 25 Feb. 2004, D-2.

Willett, Walter, M.D., Eat, Drink, and Be Healthy, Toronto: Simon and Schuster, 2001.

APPENDIX

HEALTH ASSESSMENTS

ARE YOU HEALTHY?

Record answers on the HEALTH SCORECARD (at the end of this section.)

Here is a brief rundown on measures you can do to determine your risk for heart disease, diabetes, and other diseases. These tests should be considered together before making any judgments about your health.

THESE TESTS ARE GENERAL IN NATURE, AND ARE NOT DESIGNED TO TAKE THE PLACE OF MEDICAL ADVICE.

> NOTE: Several of these tests require physical exertion. If you are over 35, a smoker, currently inactive, have a history of heart disease or other chronic medical problems, or any other concerns, check with your healthcare professional before performing the test. If at any point during these activities you experience pain, discomfort or shortness of breath, discontinue the exercise immediately.

RESTING HEART RATE: (RHR)
Your resting heart rate is the number of times your heart beats per minute when you are at rest. The best time to take your RHR is when you first wake up - before you sit up. The average American has a RHR of 72, but exercise will lower this number significantly, indicating your heart has become more efficient and requires less work to do its job.

SMOKING:
This is either a yes or no question. The reason that it is placed at the start of this inventory is because of its importance. The health risks of smoking have already been touched on. The only thing left to say is that as soon as you quit, your risk starts to tumble, and within 3-5 years, it is as low as the risk for a non-smoker. Also, seldom do you see a physically fit person who smokes. Dr. George Sheehan, the cardiologist and runner, used to say, "Give the smoker a reason to quit." An exercising body cannot tolerate smoke!

PHYSICAL ACTIVITY:
This behavior ranks right up there in importance with smoking. In fact, some authorities feel that it outranks smoking as an active person will live two years longer. More importantly, their last years on this earth will be "golden" and not "yellow." Unfortunately, based on today's health habits, the average senior will spend 5 of their last 16 years in an assisted living facility.

BODY MASS INDEX: (BMI)

In Chapter Two, you found your BMI. According to the federal government, a BMI of 25 or above puts you at an elevated risk for a number of diseases. However, this figure can be misleading. If you are fit and muscular, you may register a high BMI because muscle weighs more per pound than fat. (If you have a piece of fat that weighs 1 pound, the same size muscle would weigh 1.22 pounds, or 22% more.)

WAIST-HIP RATIO TEST:

In Chapter Two, you determined your waist-hip ratio which is an indicator for your risk of a heart attack, diabetes, stroke, high blood pressure and certain types of cancer.

BODY FAT PERCENTAGE:

This is another test that was done in Chapter Two.

BLOOD PRESSURE:

This is a measure of how open your blood vessels are. Low numbers mean that your heart doesn't have to work very hard to pump the blood through. Ideally, your blood pressure should read 120/80 or below. If your blood pressure is higher than (140 systolic or 90 diastolic), you are considered to have high blood pressure which is related to heart disease risk.

CATEGORY	SYSTOLIC	DIASTOLIC
Normal	<120	<80
Pre-Hypertension	120-130	80-89
Stage 1 Hypertension	140-159	90-99
Stage 2 Hypertension	160+	100+

BLOOD GLUCOSE:

This test measures your level of blood sugar after an overnight fast. Normal fasting blood sugar levels are less than 115 mg per deciliter (mg/dl). If your levels register between 115 mg/dl and 126 mg/dl, you have impaired fasting glucose, a risk factor for diabetes and cardiovascular disease. Fasting, plasma, and glucose levels of 126 mg/dl or above indicate diabetes. Ideally, you should strive for blood sugar levels less than 100.

BLOOD CHOLESTEROL:

Cholesterol is necessary for proper body function, but too much cholesterol in your blood leads to blockage of the arteries. Low-density lipoproteins (LDL) are known as "bad" cholesterol because they stick to the walls of the arteries, and high-density lipoproteins (HDL) are known as "good" cholesterol because they act as vacuum cleaners in your bloodstream, removing the LDL. Your LDL should be less than 130 mg/dl and your HDL greater than 40, and your total blood cholesterol level 200 mg/dl or less.

NOTE: The 2001 National Cholesterol Education Report states if you have 2 or more risk factors, i.e. age, genetic, weight, blood pressure, smoke, or have had a heart attack, that the LDL should be less than 100 and total cholesterol less than 150.

CHOLESTEROL RATIO:

Many authorities feel that of all the cholesterol numbers, this is the most important one. It is the ratio of one's LDL to HDL. Since HDL molecules remove excess cholesterol from the arteries, the more HDL you have, the less LDL and the less arterial aging you will undergo. You find this number by dividing the LDL by the HDL.

For example: If you have 150 LDL and the HDL is 50, then the ratio is 3.0. Any number above 4.0 places you in the higher risk category. If a 55 year old man had a ratio of 3.5, he would have a "RealAge" of eight years younger, or 47, whereas if his ratio was 9.0, he would have a "RealAge" of 12 years older, or 67.

CARDIOVASCULAR ENDURANCE:

This test estimates the fitness of your heart and blood vessels. You can use the one mile walk test that was in chapter 5 or one mile on a flat course. The easiest way is to go to a high school track, which is usually a quarter of a mile and do four laps (which is one mile). Start at a moderate pace but finish as fast as you can. If walking, use the chart in chapter 6. If running, use the following chart:

TIME*	RATING
7:30 minutes or less	very high endurance
7:31-8:45	high endurance
8:46-10:00	moderate endurance
10:01-11:15	low endurance
11:16 or more	very low endurance

one mile run

MUSCLE STRENGTH:

Although the strength of your muscles isn't correlated with your risk for chronic disease, your muscular fitness affects your metabolism, weight management as you age, and your ability to function well in daily life.

Upper Body Strength: Lie on the floor on your stomach, hands placed palm down next to shoulders and knees remain in contact with the floor. As you exhale, slowly raise your torso from the floor, keeping your back straight and elbows slightly bent. Slowly lower yourself to the floor and repeat as many times as you can. Refer to the chart below for your upper body strength:

NUMBER OF REPETITIONS*	LEVEL OF STRENGTH
0-9	Poor
10-19	Average
20-29	Good
30 and over	Excellent

*Persons under 35 should add 2 to each of the above repetition ranges.

Abdominal Strength Test: Lie with lower back and feet on the floor (knees bent) and arms crossed over chest. As you exhale, slowly raise shoulders off the floor as far as you can go without straining. Relax. Repeat as many times as you can. Then refer to the chart below for your abdominal strength level.

NUMBER OF REPETITIONS*	LEVEL OF STRENGTH
0-14	Poor
15-24	Average
25-34	Good
35 and over	Excellent

*Persons under 35 should add 2 to each of the above repetition ranges.

Leg Squat Test: To measure lower body strength., stand 4-8" in front of a stable chair, feet hip-width apart. Cross arms over chest, keeping back straight. Bend knees, lowering your body until your butt touches the seat. Keep heels on the floor, not letting the knees extend further than toes. Take four seconds to lower and two seconds to stand. Do as many as you can.

NUMBER OF REPETITIONS	LEVEL OF STRENGTH
25 or more	Very high strength
20-24	High strength
15-19	Moderate strength
10-14	Low strength
9 or less	Very low strength

FLEXIBILITY:

There is no single test for measuring overall flexibility. However, the trunk flexion, or "sit and reach" test, gives a good indication.

Secure a yardstick to the floor by placing a 12 inch piece of tape across at the 15 inch mark. Position yourself on the floor with the yardstick between your legs (zero toward you) and the soles of your feet about 12 inches apart and even with the tape at the 15 inch mark.

Place one hand on top of the other so the middle fingers of each hand are even. Gently lean forward along the yardstick, reaching as far as possible. Hold the position for two seconds. Note the distance. Relax, then repeat the reach two more times. Note the best distance.

AGE	WOMEN	MEN
20-29	16-21"	13-18"
30-39	15-20"	12-17"
40-49	14-19"	11-16"
50-59	13-18"	10-15"
60-69	12-17"	9-14"

If you fall within these ranges, you pass the test.

DO YOU HAVE BODY INSURANCE?

I was recently exercising at South Shore Health and Racquet Club in St. Joseph, MI, when an elderly but very spry man was "pumping" iron — a lot of it. He wore a T-shirt from the Cooper Aerobic Institute in Dallas, TX. I asked him about the shirt and he said that he's been going there for an annual fitness checkup for 25 years. He said that while the cost wasn't cheap and insurance picked up just a small portion of the cost, he decided that "If I have car and house insurance, it makes sense to also have body insurance." Too bad more of us don't have that attitude.

ON THE BACK OF THE SHIRT WAS THE FOLLOWING:

*"It's easier to maintain your health
than it is to regain it once you've lost it!"*

— Kenneth Cooper, MD

HEALTH SCORE CARD (PRE/POST)

(NOTE: Before doing the pre-test, copy this page for your post-test)

DATE:_____

TEST	SCORE	PASS/FAIL	DESIRED
Resting Heart Rate:	_____	_____	<72
Non-Smoker (Y or N)	_____	_____	YES
Physical Activity (Y or N)	_____	_____	YES
Body Mass Index	_____	_____	<26
Hip-Waist Ratio	_____	_____	<1.0-male/<.85-female
Body Fat Percentage	_____	_____	<14%-male/<20%-female
Blood Pressure	_____	_____	<130/85
Blood Glucose	_____	_____	<115
LDL Cholesterol	_____	_____	<130
HDL Cholesterol	_____	_____	>55
Total Cholesterol	_____	_____	<200
Total HDL Ratio	_____	_____	<4.0
Triglycerides	_____	_____	<120
Cardiovascular Endurance	_____	_____	walk, see chapter 6 run, see appendix
Muscle Strength			
Upper Body	_____	_____	see chart in appendix
Abdominal	_____	_____	see chart in appendix
Leg Squat	_____	_____	see chart in appendix
Flexibility	_____	_____	see chart in appendix

What are your Strengths? _____

What do you need to work on? _____

RECOMMENDED FURTHER READING

Many of the following items can be purchased from Rainbow Wellness.
For ordering information call: 269-925-3524

COOKBOOKS:

A Collection of Vegetarian Recipes, Vegetarian recipes compiled by Evelyn Kissinger.

Change Your Body One Bite at a Time, by Evelyn Kissinger, features the vegetarian lifestyle and is based on the Coronary Health Improvement Program (CHIP).

Easy Healthy Cooking, video, Evelyn Kissinger, preparing healthy meals.

Easy Healthy Shopping, video, Evelyn Kissinger, tour of grocery store.

Feast on Phytochemicals, Eve Lowry, 60 easy to prepare recipes.

Lickety-Split Meals for Health Conscious People on the Go, by Zonya Foco, RD. 3 books in one (cookbook, guide, fitness).

Ten Minute Meals – Five Minute Workouts, Robert Sweetgall and Darcy Williamson, 69 healthy meals, 22 walking workouts and 30 stretching activities.

Vegetarian Cooking, Jeanie Burke, 149 low fat vegetarian recipes with meal plans, shopping lists and gluten-free modifications. These meals have been featured on our wellness cruises.

FITNESS BOOKS: *(Authored by Rob Sweetgall)*

Pedometer Walking Book, Walking programs and journals.

Treadmill Walking, Treadmill programs and training logs.

Walk the Four Seasons, One year walking and cross training logbook.

Walking Off Weight, 14 day, 14 step lifestyle program.

Walking off Weight, Workbook that can be used with above video or separately.

FITNESS TOOLS:

DIGI WALKER KIT: Contains Digi Walker pedometer, **Pedometer Walking** book and tape measure. This book by Rob Sweetgall provides walking programs and journals.

Exerstrider Poles, Specially balanced poles and video for total body workout.

The Stick, Self massaging instrument that soothes sore muscles.

MOTIVATIONAL BOOKS and other items:

AFFIRMATIONS: www.knowitbyheart.com, Affirmations on t-shirts, cards, books.

Advice from a Tree, Journal by Ilan Shamir 800-992-4769.

Advice from a Tree Sayings, by Ilan Shamir

One Thousand Good Things Happened Today by Ilan Shamir.

Poet Tree, by Ilan Shamir

Health Care-Toons Calendar, by Jeff Haebig and Ed Fischer.

Health Care-Toons Journal, by Jeff Haebig and Ed Fischer.

Toon-Ups by Jeff Haebig and Ed Fischer.

NUTRIVISUALS: *(By Eve Lowry — these are teaching tools)*

The quality of Eve's visual displays and her scripts is unsurpassed.

"Lean Life Foods," video and recipe book.

"Lowdown on Cholesterol," 4 part video and recipe book.

"Nutrition and Your Heart," 160 slides in 4 parts with keyed scripts and cookbook.

"Phytochemicals," 100 slides, also available on CD.

"Pros: Carbs and Fats," 60 slides, script, recipes and worksheets.

ASSOCIATIONS:

American Volkssport Assn.: 1001 Pat Booker Rd., Ste. 101, Universal City, TX 78148. 210-659-2112. See the section in the walking chapter of AVA.

Human Kinetics: PO Box 5076, Champaign, IL 61825. 1-800-747-4457. Leading publisher of activity books.

Institute for Aerobic Research: 12330 Preston Rd., Dallas, TX 75230. 1-800-635-7050. Founded by Dr. Ken Cooper, the Institute provides resources on fitness.

National Senior Games: 445 N. Boulevard, Ste. 2001, Baton Rouge, LA 70802. 504-379-7337. The NSGA sponsors the National Senior Games for 50 and over.

North American Racewalking Foundation: PO Box 50312, Pasadena, CA 91115. 1-626-441-5459. The NARF provides a variety of videos and books on racewalking.

President's Council on Physical Fitness and Sport: 200 Independence Ave. SW, Room 738H, Washington DC 20201. Information on the Presidential Sports Awards for a variety of activities. (www.fitness.gov or 202-690-9000).

WELLNESS RESOURCES:

<u>Best Little Book of Wellness</u>, Dr. Donald Alsbro 269-925-3524

<u>Health Power: Health by Choice, Not Chance</u>, Dr. Hans Diehl and Aileen Ludington. 250 pages of jam-packed information on taking responsibility for our own health. The book is based on Dr. Diehl's world famous Coronary Health Improvement Program.

<u>Lifeline Health Letter</u>, (quarterly) For information on the CHIP program and related materials contact Better Health Productions, PO Box 1761, Loma Linda CA 92354.

<u>Veg News</u>, (bimonthly). Contact 415-665 NEWS or wwwvegnews.com.

<u>Vegetarian Times</u>, (monthly). 877-717-8923 or www.vegetariantimes.com.

POSSIBLE PRESENTATION TOPICS
BY DON ALSBRO

FITNESS FROM WOMB TO TOMB

SENIOR FITNESS – JUST DO IT

DEVELOPING A WELLNESS GAME PLAN

DUMP YOUR PLUMP™

WORK-SITE WELLNESS PROGRAMS

THE FUTURE OF WELLNESS

THE FUTURE OF HEALTH AND PHYSICAL EDUCATION

TAKE THE WELLNESS ROAD

WELLNESS CRUISES

FOR BOOKINGS CONTACT

Donald E. Alsbro, Ed.D., CHES

942 Sierra Drive

Benton Harbor, MI 49022

269-925-3524

dealsbro@sbcglobal.net

www.dumpyourplump.com

OTHER BOOKS BY THIS AUTHOR
THE "DUMP YOUR PLUMP™" CONTEST MANUAL
First edition: 1988, Revisions: 1992, 1995

THE BEST LITTLE BOOK OF WELLNESS,
First edition: 1998; Second edition (Revised): 2000,
Third edition: (Revised) 2002

CRUISE TESTIMONIALS

"Great trip and very well organized! Thank you." — Tony and Bonnie Korican, Stevensville, MI

"First cruise – celebrated our 50th anniversary – Ken turned 75 and we had FUN! I brought a pedometer and we walked 55 miles during cruise week. I did not gain any weight. For some years, I've racked my brain to get Ken enthusiastic about travel. You talked me into the cruise and Ken loved it – So health holding we have signed up for Alaska in June and the Western Caribbean in Feb. Thanks for all you both (Don and Sharon) do to make "smooth sailing" for an old couple." — Pat and Ken Morrison, Berrien Springs, MI

"The people were all very friendly. The food was great. The scenery was beautiful and the classes were educational." — Betty Edinborough, Coloma, MI

"Thanks so much for all your have done to put this fantastic experience together. We had a great time, learned so much and made many new and interesting friends." — Jackie Goode, Crest Hill, IL

"Being with friends and making new friends. The best vacation we've ever had. It makes it a vacation with a purpose! Thanks for getting us in at the last minute." — Kristy Plata, Lindsay, CA

"The speakers, the food, and the life changing information. Ate like a pig and lost four pounds." — Kathryn Grimm, Los Angeles, CA

"So many things! Meeting old friends and making new friends. I really appreciated 'the feeding of the soul' as well as the intellect and exercise information." — Lucy Kieft, Grand Rapids, MI

"Overall, I had a blast. The entire vacation was a big party! Just what I wanted." — Barb Helgerson, Madison, WI

"This was our second wellness cruise. Things we enjoyed were the friendships formed, morning walks, exercise room, Jacuzzi, sauna and the variety of classes to select from. The ability to relax, yet enjoy ourselves with the many opportunities on the boat will always be remembered." — John and Kathy Campbell, Glendale AZ

"The wellness topics were diverse and very interesting. The presenters were well prepared and very professional. I commend Don Alsbro on his commitment to health and wellness. It was a wonderful cruise and my best vacation!" — Jacqueline Owen, Cleveland OH

OTHER WELLNESS OPPORTUNITIES

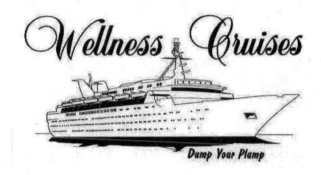

Dr. Alsbro organizes
"WELLNESS TRAVEL"

CRUISES to Eastern and Western CARIBBEAN, ALASKA, ETC. and other "WELLNESS TRIPS"

FEATURING

Nationally Known Health and Wellness Experts in:

- ◆ **FITNESS ACTIVITIES**
- ◆ **WORKSHOPS**
- ◆ **ENTERTAINING HEALTH SESSIONS**
- ◆ **FUN!!!!!!!!**

Prices start at $995.00!
For information on our next trip, contact:
Dr. Don Alsbro at 1-800-67PLUMP.
www.wellnesscruise.org/

Shape Up!

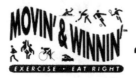

Join "Movin' & Winnin'®" "Spring Training"

"DUMP YOUR PLUMP®"

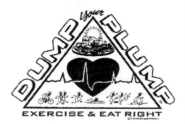

EXERCISE & EAT RIGHT

National Internet Weight-Loss and Fitness Contests

for

Teams from Businesses, Organizations, Friends, Etc.

Have Fun!

Form a team where you work
- *4 – 10 members per team*

Set a weight-loss goal of 0-20 lbs.
- *Weekly weigh-ins at your work place*

Develop new health habits
- *Special programs and health tests*
- *Daily aerobic exercise*
- *Program manual and newsletters*
- *Prizes for weight loss, exercise and best team name*

♦ **Web page for EACH Team**

♦ **Chat room with experts and fellow contestants**

♦ **Compete locally and nationally**

For more information and to sign up, Call: Don Alsbro at (269) 925-3524 or Email: dealsbro@sbcglobal.net or go to: www.dumpyourplump.com

GIVE YOUR FRIENDS AND FAMILY
THE GIFT OF A LIFETIME

To purchase additional copies of this book fill out the information below and send the form, along with check made payable to Rainbow Wellness (or provide credit card information), to the address below.

Ship-to Name_____

Address_____

City _____ State _____ Zip _____

Phone_____ e-Mail_____

Credit Card #_____

Expiration Date _____

Is the person purchasing the book also the recipient? _____ Y_____N

If no, what is the purchaser's name? _____

Phone_____

Would you like the book autographed? _____ Y_____N

If yes, please indicate recipient's name _____

PRICE		
1-2: $12.95 ea.	3+: $10.95 ea.	
SHIPPING		
1-2: $5.00	3+: Add 10%	
SALES TAX: MI Residents +6%		
TOTAL		

SUBMIT ORDER TO:
Rainbow Wellness, Inc.
942 Sierra Drive
Benton Harbor, MI 49022

Please allow 2-3 weeks for delivery.

NOTES

NOTES